Untold Stories of Disablement and Displacement

Praise for this book

'With the utmost respect, empathy, and compassion using the art of storytelling and stimulating research Dr. Dada offers an intellectual and heartfelt captivating and critical examination of a vital intersection that the international community, disability advocates and governments which have ratified the UN Convention on the Rights of Persons with Disabilities or pledge to uphold human rights, must take serious note of. This passionate book incites a moral courage to recognize where commitments to refugees and people seeking asylum, as well as responsibilities to the disability community, are falling short and calls upon the promise that is Canada, to do better. Furthermore, this masterpiece inspires a more profound and equitable approach to the social and human rights model of disability inclusion. If anything it is a guide to better serve humanity in all its diversity.'

Cara E. Yar Khan, Disability advocate and
United Nations humanitarian

'Sukaina Dada is a much-needed new voice on disability and migration. She has shown us the incredible power of story telling, bringing to life the diverse and complex stories of Syrian refugees and in doing so she reminds us of our shared humanity and social responsibility for populations marginalized through racism, disablement, and migration. This book should be read by anyone who is trying to change how we understand and respond to the global migrant crisis.'

Professor Marina Morrow, Critical Disability Studies,
York University

Untold Stories of Disablement and Displacement
Syrian refugees in Canada

Sukaina Dada

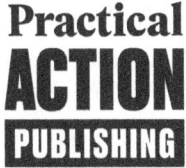

Practical Action Publishing Ltd
25 Albert Street, Rugby,
Warwickshire, CV21 2SD, UK
www.practicalactionpublishing.com

© Sukaina Dada 2025

The author has asserted their right under the Copyright, Designs and Patents Act 1988 to be identified as author of this work.

All rights reserved. No part of this publication may be reprinted or reproduced or utilized in any form or by any electronic, mechanical, or other means, now known or hereafter invented, including photocopying and recording, or in any information storage or retrieval system, without the written permission of the publishers.

Product or corporate names may be trademarks or registered trademarks, and are used only for identification and explanation without intent to infringe.

A catalogue record for this book is available from the British Library.

A catalogue record for this book has been requested from the Library of Congress.

ISBN 978-1-78853-403-1 Paperback
ISBN 978-1-78853-405-5 Electronic book

Citation: Dada, S., (2025) *Untold Stories of Disablement and Displacement: Syrian refugees in Canada,* Rugby, UK: Practical Action Publishing
http://doi.org/10.3362/9781788534055

Since 1974, Practical Action Publishing has published and disseminated books and information in support of international development work throughout the world.

Practical Action Publishing is a trading name of Practical Action Publishing Ltd (Company Reg. No. 1159018), the wholly owned publishing company of Practical Action. Practical Action Publishing trades only in support of its parent charity objectives and any profits are covenanted back to Practical Action (Charity Reg. No. 247257, Group VAT Registration No. 880 9924 76).

The views and opinions in this publication are those of the author and do not represent those of Practical Action Publishing Ltd or its parent charity Practical Action.

Reasonable efforts have been made to publish reliable data and information, but the author and publisher cannot assume responsibility for the validity of all materials or for the consequences of their use.

Cover design by: Katarzyna Markowska, Practical Action Publishing Typeset by vPrompt eServices, India

The manufacturer's authorised representative in the EU for product safety is Lightning Source France, 1 Av. Johannes Gutenberg, 78310 Maurepas, France.
compliance@lightningsource.fr

To Imraan,
My love and best friend, thank you for being there
every step of the way.

To Hamzah and Aayah,
My babies. Speak your truth – your story always matters.

To Fatema, Akila, Hawa, Faisal, and Fahad,
My confidants and cheerleaders. Your support means everything.

To Mom and Dad,
Your sacrifices and encouragement shaped who I am today.

To my beautiful baby Aasiyah Haleema,
May we be reunited one day.
May Allah Almighty shower His infinite mercy upon you.
Ameen.

Contents

Acknowledgements	ix
About the author	x

1. Introduction	1
Introducing my story	1
The storytellers	5
A crisis devoid of urgency	11
Private sponsorship	12
A global pandemic	15
Disability defined	18
2. The power of stories	21
The danger of the single story	22
The dominant narrative: welcoming refugees in Canada	24
3. Collecting the stories	31
Limitations to collecting and sharing stories	34
Stories unveiled amidst chaos	35
4. Theoretical underpinnings	37
Models of disability	37
Transnational model of disability	44
Citizenship	47
Othering the other	49
Intersectional oppressions	51
5. Sharing real-life stories	57
Stories of disablement	57
Stories of a disabling Syria	61
Stories of difficult journeys	64
Stories of trauma	68
Stories of Canadian struggles	72
Stories of economic and social conditions	75
Stories of a pandemic survival	80
Stories of securing rights	85
Stories of gratitude	89
Stories of inclusion	92
Stories of advocacy	96

6. Listening to our stories 103
   Advocacy to action 108

7. Final reflections 113
   The disablement of Gaza 115

References 119
Index 139

Acknowledgements

This book is a revised version of my 2022 PhD study. I would like to acknowledge the talented and brave Dr. Rachel da Silveira Gorman for helping me find my voice, encouraging me to be intentional in my work, and not letting me shy away from critical issues.

I would like to acknowledge the participants in the study for their time, energy, and expertise and for trusting me with their stories.

I would like to acknowledge and thank my team at SMILE Canada – Support Services who work every day to break down barriers.

About the author

Dr. Sukaina Dada has dedicated over 16 years to advancing the health and well-being of children, with a particular emphasis on addressing the health disparities faced by racialized and newcomer children with disabilities. A passionate advocate for the protection of children's rights worldwide, she has consistently worked to ensure that vulnerable children receive the care and support they are entitled to. Dr. Dada is a paediatric occupational therapist with extensive experience working with children and youth with disabilities in diverse community and healthcare settings. As the founder and CEO of SMILE Canada – Support Services, a Canadian charity, Dr. Dada spearheads initiatives aimed at supporting newcomer children and youth with disabilities and their families. Her grassroots efforts have had a profound impact on policy, particularly in advocating for anti-racism, safer spaces, and culturally responsive support and resources.

Dr. Dada holds a PhD in Critical Disability Studies from the School of Health Policy and Management at York University, where her research focused on the intersection of displacement and disability. She recently completed a visiting postdoctoral fellowship at York University, where she helped developed an artificial intelligence-based search engine to support global disability advocates, in collaboration with the UNCRPD Secretariat. In recognition of her outstanding contributions, Dr. Dada has been honoured with several prestigious awards, including being named a finalist for the RBC Women of the Year Award. She has also received the McMaster Arch Alumni Award and the McMaster University Distinguished Alumni Award in Rehabilitation Science.

CHAPTER 1
Introduction

Introducing my story

My core values, fundamental principles, and critical knowledge come from the stories I grew up on. They were not made-up fables or exaggerated tales. They formed my life lessons, my life truths. The stories of my father dropping out of school at the age of six, working countless odd jobs to support his family, and never again receiving any formal education. The stories of my mother and her family escaping dangerous conditions during the Zanzibar revolution as thousands of Arab, Iranian, and South Asian families were expelled from the Island (Bakari, 2001). The stories of my maternal great-grandmother, who lost 10 of her 11 children before she passed away – through poverty, violence, and medical institutionalization. I heard stories of migration, conflict, and community. They were stories of pain and hardship and stories of strength and resilience. My parents' and grandparents' stories were of diaspora. They wove into transnational narratives of colonialism and settler colonialism.

These stories taught me about my identity, family, culture, and faith and helped shape my own story. As a Muslim woman of colour, growing up in Kitchener, Ontario, my central story became one of assimilation and enforced gratitude. I did not endure the economic or social hardships my parents did. My story was different. Even though I had the benefit of going to publicly funded schools, accessing universal healthcare and social services, and having the economic security of my parents, it became apparent to me that the heroes in the dominant stories that surrounded me were different from the ones in my life story. Be it in media, literature, education, or social policy, the dominant stories did not reflect families who looked like or sounded like mine.

After high school, this dominant narrative became more evident when my younger cousin Muhammad migrated to Canada from Tanzania. I was always fond of Muhammad; he was kind and gentle, and his laughter was contagious. Muhammad was diagnosed with cerebral palsy shortly after he arrived; the doctors said he could not see, hear, walk, or talk. They spoke about how he would never be independent and that he may only experience involuntary movement. 'It is not clear what he actually understands', the neurologist bluntly said as Muhammad squirmed in my lap, giggling every time my hands gently crossed his belly. The doctors provided pamphlets of paediatric long-term care facilities where we could leave him, as the caregiver burden may be 'too much to handle'. While they were quick to dismiss Muhammad's life, and our family's culture, we knew he could love and would be loved. As we navigated through the healthcare and social services sectors, I observed the numerous barriers Muhammad faced; it was not only his disability, but the colour of his skin, his Muslim name, his mother's hijab, his immigration status, and so on. Time and time again, I witnessed healthcare workers, service providers, and educators ignore his life story.

Upon graduating from university, I set out to work with children with disabilities and pursued a master's degree in occupational therapy. As I worked with clients from different racialized communities, it became apparent that stories of displacement and disablement were rarely acknowledged. I found this both ironic and harmful, as the profession of occupational therapy seeks to identify barriers to meaningful occupation, social participation, and health and well-being by considering one's whole story (Sakellariou and Pollard, 2016). As an occupational therapist, I learned about client-centred and family-centred care, but the stories of the newcomer families coming into the clinic where I worked were largely disregarded. As part of the occupational therapy programme, I conducted a study that examined the lived experiences of Muslim children with disabilities and their families in Canada. The collective narratives of oppression experienced by the participants led me to form SMILE Canada – Support Services (SMILE), a registered Canadian charity intended to address the barriers that racialized and newcomer children with disabilities and their families face in Canada, specifically from under-served and under-represented communities. Through my clinical work and my experiences at SMILE, I encountered many families who shared their struggles with feeling isolated and marginalized in community spaces. They reported both explicit and implicit instances of xenophobia, Islamophobia, racism, and ableism within healthcare settings. Additionally, they faced challenges in accessing vital educational resources and had difficulty navigating social and healthcare services.

After several years of practicing as an occupational therapist, I realized that I wanted to pursue further studies to examine the critical relationship of disablement and displacement, which led me to the PhD study that informed this book. In 2017, when the Syrian war was gaining more international attention, the Canadian government responded by opening the borders to Syrian refugees. I never felt prouder to be Canadian than when Prime Minister Justin Trudeau publicly stated on X that Canada will accept Muslims and Arabs fleeing persecution (Hughes, 2019). I was relieved to read the Prime Minister's response to the millions of displaced Syrians. I was in the process of moving back to Canada from the United States following then-president Donald Trump's unexpected election victory. Trudeau's response was immeasurably different from the racist, xenophobic, and Islamophobic content that Trump spewed daily on US television networks and social media outlets, making Canada's public commitment even more special.

However, my excitement was quickly overcome with disappointment. Following the infamous public tweet, I began to meet Syrian children with disabilities through my grassroots work at SMILE. One day, I received a phone call that made me really question the dominant narrative that surrounded Canada's response to the Syrian refugee crisis – the narrative that was plastered across local and international headlines, reiterating Canada as a hero welcoming Syrian refugees while neighbouring countries rejected them. A principal of a Toronto public school called me regarding a 'disruptive' and 'noncompliant' disabled student who could not remain in his current classroom for the following reasons: 1) the child did not know how to use basic classroom tools; 2) he had difficulty interacting with other children; and 3) every time the bell rang, he hid under the desk with his head between his legs, screaming and rocking back and forth. Before I had a chance to respond with what I thought would be a logical explanation for why a child who recently sought asylum in Canada from a refugee camp escaping armed conflict was having difficulty adjusting to his new school environment, the principal responded, 'I know what you are going to say. He came from a war-torn country, but how long will we use that as an excuse?' The principal's comments, while shocking, reflect the narrative that disabled refugees now in Canada must forget their stories formed through their experiences and oppressions. They must quickly get over their trauma and be grateful for their chance at a new life.

As the months went by, I worked with many Syrian families and, soon, those feel-good comments by government officials and media images of Syrian refugees sipping Tim Hortons coffee and wearing Canada Goose jackets faded into the background. I began to see the many systemic barriers that impact disabled refugees in Canada. While many Canadians supported the resettlement of Syrian refugees in Canada, I could not help but question whether we were welcoming refugees with open arms as portrayed in the media. Were we only accepting of the ideal refugee – the non-disabled, educated one who was ready to get into the workforce and 'give back'? I met so many families struggling to be included in public spaces, who were met with discrimination and who were denied basic rights and services, but these were not the families I saw on television or read about in the paper. The stories we heard on the news were painted over with a brush of assimilation and an erasure of trauma. The notes of pain, fear, and hardship were removed from the narratives of the very people who sought refuge in Canada.

As I further explored the rights of disabled refugees in Canada, I found a striking absence of information on the complex relationship between displacement and disability. Disabled persons continue to be among the most exposed and excluded groups in any displaced society (Women's Refugee Committee, 2013). Disabled refugees are ignored within humanitarian spheres, including programs designed to support displaced persons (Crock et al., 2017). They are often overlooked in the planning of emergency healthcare services (Kett & Van Ommeren, 2009; Mirza, 2011) and are at a higher risk of physical and sexual abuse, exploitation, abandonment, and death during conflicts and national emergencies (Crock et al., 2017). Many disabled refugees have experienced torture, trauma, and malnutrition (Taleb et al., 2015). Furthermore, many refugees do not report disabilities for fear of being left behind or enduring human rights abuses (Bradley & Tawfiq, 2006).

Displacement has a direct correlation with disablement, so how is such a powerful intersection left out of critical conversations on human rights, social justice, and structural and social determinants of health and disability? The intersection of disablement and displacement is rarely examined in public forums, academic discourse, or within social policies. I was drawn to a quote by feminist scholar Judith Butler, who asked, '[w]hich bodies matter, and which bodies are yet to emerge as critical matters of concern?' (Butler, 1993, p. 4). While Butler posed this question in the context of gender equality, it is correspondingly salient as a concern for disabled refugees: do their stories matter? Are they yet to transpire as worthy of critical attention? Research around disabled refugees, while slim, has primarily been quantitative, highlighting the numbers of people disabled and displaced, not their experiences (Elder, 2015). We frequently hear the statistics of the number of refugees 'let into' Canada, but behind the figures are real stories of disabled persons – forced to evacuate their homes and leave behind their familiar surroundings due to structural violence, extreme poverty, and persecution. Once settled, their stories are overlooked.

This book is my attempt to uncover and record some of the authentic and unexamined narratives of disabled refugees and their families, and to build on the disruption in disability studies grounded in colonial whiteness, already shaken by the likes of Gorman (2005, 2007, 2016, 2018), Erevelles (2002, 2011, 2014), Razack (1998, 2013), Puar (2017), and Dossa (2009, 2013), amongst others. I hope to offer others even a glimpse of the profound impact I experienced while listening to the narratives of disablement and displacement.

This research contributes a unique and vital perspective to academic literature by challenging and disrupting the dominant narrative around disabled refugees, a narrative which overshadows spaces in academia, media, and popular culture and that strategically segregates disablement from displacement. Although the stories shared by participants might have been challenging to recount, storytelling and sharing truths is an act capable of challenging prevailing narratives and catalysing social change by unveiling those truths (Dossa, 2013, p. 103).

The storytellers

Participant stories reflect both dominant national and transnational narratives around disablement and displacement. I interviewed 10 Syrian families to provide a glimpse into the narratives of disabled refugees and the material and social conditions that shape their experiences. The stories of these 10 families led to 11 themes derived from real-life stories.

Prior to each interview, the purpose of the study and the research questions were discussed with the potential participants for transparency. The narrative research method does not impose strict measures about the number of questions posed during an interview, nor does it dictate which questions must be answered. Instead, the process allows the stories to ebb and flow as the participant narrates. Employing a semi-structured interview guide, inspired by DeJonckheere and Vaughn (2019) and Walliman (2006), I encouraged participants to narrate their experiences in their own words. Open-ended questions, as highlighted by Pope and Mays (2006) and Dossa (2009), were used to capture the richness of these real-life experiences, recognizing that complex narratives cannot be reduced to simple data.

I began each conversation by saying, 'We all have a story, and today, I would like to know about your story'. All participants consented to the use of pseudonyms and the removal of identifying information. The pseudonyms chosen were culturally relevant, using common Arabic names from Syria and its surrounding regions. To further protect anonymity, pseudonyms were also employed for individuals who supported and worked with the participants.

I share a brief profile of each participant, and their family below based off the detailed accounts they shared with me. These profiles are an insufficient introduction to the participants I interacted with. I could write chapters about the storied lives of each person who shared their narratives with me. Their conversations have stuck with me in an unexpected way and have challenged me to further examine disablement and displacement through non-dominant stories. As I combed through the detailed transcripts of the stories, themes stood out in a way that underscored how the participants' stories were interwoven. I never discussed the participants' stories or profiles with each other. I never disclosed whom else I interviewed and never shared any participant information with the other families, but it was as though participants shared their stories with one another ahead of time. Their stories were distinct yet similar. They were individual yet shared. Their fears, challenges, hopes for their children, and desire for a better future were echoed with a collective voice.

Marwa

Marwa and her siblings were born and raised in a small village in Syria. Marwa got married and had her first child during her teenage years. In her town, it was common for girls to marry at 15 or 16 years of age and have children early on, then stay home to care for their families. Very few girls would continue post-secondary education or work outside the home. However, Marwa was keen on pursuing a professional career, but she did not have educational opportunities. Marwa described education as 'life'. She wanted to attend graduation and walk across a stage to receive a diploma. She heard about it from her friends and had seen clips of graduation ceremonies in movies. When the war broke out, Marwa fled Syria with her husband and disabled children. When she learned about the possibility of seeking refuge in Canada, she first thought about how her children could be formally educated and have more opportunities to succeed professionally. Marwa applied through different avenues to come to Canada. After months of trying, she was contacted by a private Muslim charitable organization that assisted her with private refugee sponsorship. Now living in Canada, Marwa and her husband pursue adult education classes while maintaining full-time employment to make ends meet.

Amal

Amal and her husband, Yusuf, were born and raised in Damascus, and both lived with physical disabilities for most of their lives. Amal faced numerous challenges as a disabled person, including social exclusion, lack of support in school, obstacles to adequate employment, and environmental barriers to accessing professional spaces due to her wheelchair use. When the situation in Syria became unbearable, and Amal's family home and business were destroyed, she fled to a refugee camp in Jordan, hoping for a better life for her family, including her disabled child. However, life in the refugee camp was even worse than expected, with unsanitary, dangerous, and inaccessible conditions. Amal and her family could not leave the refugee camp freely due to the rough terrains that surrounded the camp. They were confined to a small space all day and night. They could not send their children to school, nor could they obtain employment. After a few years, Amal and her family were resettled through the Blended Visa Office-Referred (BVOR) programme in Canada.

Halima

Halima was born and raised in a bustling Syrian metropolis. She met Ahmed in college and their bond quickly led to marriage and the arrival of their first child. Halima described her life to be one full of hope. She had a bright professional future ahead of her. She and her husband dreamed of pursuing further education and growing their family business. However, the outbreak of war shattered their dreams, prompting a hasty evacuation to Egypt with their children. Though faced with the challenges of raising children with developmental delays in an unknown environment, Halima remained resolute in her commitment to their well-being, ensuring a nurturing and secure environment throughout her displacement journey. Recognizing the promising prospects for disabled children in Canada, Halima made the decision to seek asylum through the private sponsorship programme. Now settled with her husband and children, she is determined to build a brighter future in her newfound home.

Muhammad

Muhammad fondly recalls his upbringing in a close-knit Syrian town where everyone was like one big family. Muhammad devoted himself wholeheartedly to both his career and family. He married young and became a father to children who faced challenges communicating with others and keeping up with their peers in school. When the war broke out, Muhammad and his family sought refuge in Jordan, where they stayed for a few challenging years marked by the struggle to secure employment and support for their disabled children. Muhammad's cousin, who was living in Canada at the time, encouraged him to apply for refuge through the United Nations refugee process. Following a successful application, Muhammad and his loved ones were granted asylum and eventually arrived in Canada, eager to embark on a new chapter in their lives.

Hajra

Hajra was born in a small town in Syria. She married immediately after high school and had her first child shortly afterwards. When she fled Syria to Lebanon, she learned about Canada's private sponsorship programme for Syrian refugees. Hajra's children had multiple disabilities and had significant difficulties communicating, socializing, and learning in school, and Hajra wanted them to get the medical and educational support they required. Complicating matters further, her husband's inability to join them in Canada, due to his commitment to supporting relatives denied refugee status, left Hajra assuming the role of a single mother upon their arrival in Canada. Hajra and her children were privately sponsored. Once the sponsorship support ran dry, Hajra faced difficulties caring for her family. With financial responsibilities resting solely on her shoulders, she faces the daunting task of providing for her family without the aid of relatives or sufficient social and financial support.

Hassan

Hassan described his life in Syria before the war as a life that made him proud. He was a reputable and talented business owner and a loving family man. Hassan faced the challenges of nurturing three children with delays in communication, mobility, and learning, sparing no effort in providing them with additional tutoring and therapies to ensure they received the necessary support. However, the eruption of armed conflict shattered his world, forcing him to abandon everything he held dear. Witnessing the devastation of his neighbourhood and the loss of countless friends and relatives, Hassan's paramount concern became the safety of his family. Seeking refuge in Egypt, he welcomed a fourth child, who was also born with a disability. Determined to secure a safer future for his family, Hassan sought asylum in Canada through the United Nations refugee process. Now settled, he shoulders the responsibility of caring for his wife, who battles a chronic health condition, alongside their disabled children. With no familial or social support network in Canada, Hassan faces the challenge of maintaining employment while fulfilling his caretaking duties.

Muna

Muna's life in Syria was severely challenging from a young age. She struggled with poverty her entire life and caring for a disabled child was difficult with the many social, economic, and political changes in Syria. The outbreak of war plunged her into a nightmare, where the fear of losing a child became a haunting reality as she witnessed the loss of loved ones, including several children in her community. Seeking refuge from the devastation, Muna fled Syria with her family and sought refuge in Jordan. Muna applied for asylum in Canada with her children through the United Nations refugee process. In Canada, Muna assumes the role of a stay-at-home mum. She wants her children to receive a quality education so that they will have economic opportunities she was not afforded.

Sarah

Sarah's narrative unfolded with the recounting of a harrowing forced marriage to a relative. She shared how complicated her pregnancies were and described how she struggled to get adequate healthcare in Syria. Amidst these trials, she grappled with the additional burden of her family's lack of acceptance and understanding of her children's disabilities. The outbreak of war only served to compound the complexities of her marital situation, leaving her torn between meeting her own needs and those of her children. Fleeing the turmoil, Sarah embarked on a migration journey with her children and then-partner to Lebanon, where she initiated the arduous process of seeking refuge through the United Nations. Now, in Canada, Sarah is a single mum and the sole provider and advocate for her children.

Omar

Once the war erupted in Syria, Omar and his family hastily fled, seeking refuge in Jordan. There, Omar advocated tirelessly to get his child medical attention and educational support. With his son's medical condition serving as the impetus, Omar navigated the United Nations refugee process to apply for resettlement in Canada, citing exceptional humanitarian circumstances. After a few years of anticipation, Omar, along with his wife and children, finally arrived in their new home. However, settling into life in Canada presented its own challenges for Omar, particularly concerning his personal health needs. Despite his sincere desire to attain full-time, meaningful employment, he grapples with the difficult balance of managing work commitments alongside his long-term health condition and his familial responsibilities.

Dalia

Dalia, the eldest participant in the study, faced the upheaval of war head-on, fleeing Syria alongside her partner Mahmoud and their adult children to find refuge in Egypt. While in Egypt, Dalia was split up from her children who were eligible to migrate to Europe for their professional careers. However, Dalia and Mahmoud were rejected from seeking asylum in Europe due to their age, lack of education and professional careers, and their documented disabilities. After some time, Dalia and her husband applied for refuge in Canada through the United Nations refugee process and were granted asylum. Yet, the path to safety came with a high cost, as Dalia now finds herself alone in Canada with Mahmoud, separated from her children and grappling with the challenges of living with disabilities without any caregiver support.

Insights from key advocates

In addition to the in-depth interviews with the above storytellers, it was imperative to gain insight into the experiences of settlement workers and private sponsors dedicated to supporting and advocating for disabled Syrian refugees. I draw upon the perspectives of three private sponsors – Naima, Najma, and Jahan – as well as the vital insights provided by two seasoned settlement workers, Salma and Yasmine. Additionally, I include personal testimony from my sister, Fatema, who volunteered at a Syrian refugee camp on the island of Leros, Greece, several years ago. Her firsthand account sheds light on the unique challenges faced by displaced Syrians with disabilities.

A crisis devoid of urgency

While the term 'Syrian refugee crisis' has gained international popularity over the years, it is a polished umbrella term highlighting the displacement of millions who have been uprooted by the 2011 conflict in Syria and the ongoing proxy wars fought in surrounding areas (UNHCR, 2024a). This term has become diluted and devoid of urgency. The Syrian refugee crisis has resulted in over half of the Syrian population being displaced, with approximately 25 per cent of them living with disabilities (Humanity and Inclusion, 2015; UNHCR, 2018). By March 2021, the numbers were staggering, with approximately 6.6 million Syrians externally displaced and another 7.2 million internally displaced (UNHCR, 2024a). Of those who sought refuge outside Syria, more than 75 per cent fled to neighbouring countries like Lebanon, Türkiye, Jordan, and Egypt (UNHCR, 2024a). This forced displacement stems from a complex interplay of domestic and international factors, including the destabilization of Syria triggered by the 2003 US invasion of Iraq, the Arab Spring uprisings, and the subsequent Syrian civil war (Bakke and Kuypers, 2016; Bose, 2020). The ongoing violence, environmental destruction, and collapse of health and education systems in Syria continues to drive families into disablement and displacement. The enormity of the Syrian refugee crisis led to the Canadian government's 'Operation Syrian Refugees' initiative in November 2015 to settle 25,000 Syrian refugees across Canada over 12 months (Government of Canada, 2020a). Since then, the resettlement efforts have steadily increased, reaching over 44,000 individuals (Government of Canada, 2024) Canada has prioritized the resettlement of vulnerable families, including those with disabled family members, and with nearly half of the resettled individuals being under the age of 15 (Houle, 2019; UNHCR, 2020; Bose, 2020).

Private sponsorship

Although not a new concept in Canada, the private refugee sponsorship programme garnered international recognition for its response to the Syrian refugee crisis (Kaida et al., 2020). Originating in the late 1970s, the Canadian government initiated this once-unique private sponsorship programme to respond to the humanitarian crisis in China (Lanphier, 2003; Labman, 2016). Over time, the programme evolved, with revisions that allowed community groups such as faith-based and cultural groups, as well as groups of five individuals (G5), and sponsorship agreement holders (SAH), which include organizations that have signed agreements with the Government of Canada to support refugees collectively for approximately one year (UNHCR, 2022). These groups must demonstrate both the willingness and financial ability to sponsor refugees. Sponsors bear the entire cost of resettlement, including essential expenses such as housing, furniture, clothing, and transportation, with the sponsorship group often raising additional funds to support refugees financially (Kamran, 2023). Furthermore, private sponsors provide social and emotional support and help families traverse the complex health, educational, and social service systems (Government of Canada, 2020a). While initially, private sponsorship was secondary to government-sponsored refugees, by 2016, nearly half of all Syrian refugees were brought to Canada through private sponsorship (Government of Canada, 2016; UNHCR, 2022). According to a sponsorship cost table provided by Immigration, Refugees and Citizenship Canada, sponsoring a family of five is estimated to cost $35,500 per year (RSTP, 2018). Since 1979, Canadian citizens have privately sponsored over 327,000 refugees (UNHCR, 2022). While private sponsorship appears to be an innovative approach to increasing the number of refugees in Canada, the programme's voluntary nature poses significant challenges, as private sponsors often bear increased responsibilities with fewer resources than the government. Chris Alexander, Minister of Immigration, Refugees and Citizenship of Canada (2013–2015) addressed concerns from the media regarding the responsibilities of private sponsors with the following statement: 'Hundreds of private sponsorship opportunities remain. We encourage sponsorship agreement holders to do their part to help displaced Syrians'. This statement strongly urged private sponsors to act, which may have, at least in part, shifted some responsibility for supporting refugees away from the government (Labman, 2016, p. 8). This voluntary responsibility can be burdensome for individuals who may lack the capacity, willingness, or ability to fulfil their sponsorship duties, leaving refugees in precarious situations.

Among the participants I interviewed, their paths to Canada varied, with the majority arriving through the Government-Assisted Refugee (GAR) programme, others through the BVOR programme, and some via private sponsorship. The BVOR programme stands out as a cost-sharing initiative where both the government and private sponsors shoulder the financial responsibilities of the sponsored refugees (Haugen, 2019). Of the three participants I interviewed who had support from private sponsors and volunteers, two reported receiving substantial assistance upon their arrival and were provided with the necessary resources to ease their transition into Canadian life. Marwa shared that their private sponsor had gone 'above and beyond' to help her during the challenging process of resettlement. Halima reported wanting to continue the same level of support her family received when they first arrived and shared how the year was extremely challenging and went by too quickly. Once the year passed, her sponsor lost touch with her, and she felt neglected. Amal reported feeling abandoned by the very people who signed up to care for her and her family:

> I didn't know any resources, and I lived in a small community, I came to the unknown and I think it wasn't fair that I came through private sponsorship – not like other people who came and were given information on where to go or what to do.

Naima, a private sponsorship volunteer whom I interviewed, shed light on the initial framing of the BVOR programme, which was presented as an avenue for financially supporting refugees for six months and then providing social and emotional support for an additional six months under the guidance of the Canadian government (IRCC, 2022). However, the reality for Naima and her colleagues was quite different, as they discovered that very little assistance was forthcoming. 'What we did not anticipate is the lack of guidance', she explained. 'We undertook this [sponsorship] because we ourselves arrived in Canada as refugees. We wanted to extend a helping hand, and it felt gratifying to be able to support others on their journey.' Naima went on to describe how private sponsorship did not align with her expectations; instead, it introduced a power dynamic that positioned the refugee family as inferior. 'It fell upon us, the sponsors, to either allocate the funds provided to the families or to assist them by purchasing necessary items and guiding them through the process. This placed us in a very challenging position.' When the allocated funding ran dry, Naima and her fellow community members involved in the sponsorship had to rely heavily on personal funds and resources to continue supporting the families. Naima spoke of the dominant narrative of private sponsorship and how it was a false narrative that the government would be there 'every step of the way'. In recent years, private sponsors have had to do more for families with less funding (Labman, 2016). While the private sponsorship model has no doubt allowed private citizens to support displaced persons seeking refuge in Canada, it is concerning that it has become the dominant method of resettling in Canada for Syrian refugees (CCR, 2017). With fewer funds, more commitment, and less guidance and oversight, private sponsors may be unable to provide culturally responsive, adequate, and safe support.

A global pandemic

In January 2020, my research on disablement and displacement took an unexpected turn with the emergence of the novel coronavirus, COVID-19, as reported by the World Health Organization (WHO, 2021). Within weeks, this fatal virus rapidly spread across the globe. By 2021, over 335 million confirmed cases and more than 5 million deaths had been reported worldwide (Worldometer, 2021).

At the onset of the COVID-19 outbreak, Syria's healthcare system was already fragile due to years of armed conflict and inadequate resources, and over 60 per cent of Syria's population required humanitarian assistance. Since 2020, the living situation in Syria deteriorated significantly due to the spread of the pandemic. Recognizing the urgency of the situation, on 23 March 2020, Antonio Guterres, the UN Secretary-General, issued an international plea calling for a global ceasefire: 'Our world faces a common enemy: COVID-19. The virus does not care about nationality or ethnicity, faction, or faith. It attacks all, relentlessly. Meanwhile, armed conflict rages around the world. The most vulnerable – women and children, people with disabilities, the marginalized and the displaced – pay the highest price' (UNICEF, 2020).

The government policies and measures implemented to mitigate the spread of the COVID-19 virus posed significant challenges for displaced persons seeking refuge in host countries. By April 2020, over 160 countries had either partially or entirely closed their borders (UNHCR, 2021b), turning away refugees, compelling them to return to the dangerous and uninhabitable environments they had fled. Additionally, many search and rescue operations in the

Mediterranean that were vital for protecting refugees fleeing by boat were suspended due to the pandemic's impact (Kluge et al., 2020). Following a statement around the difficult living conditions refugees endured, Tedros Adhanom Ghebreyesus, the Director-General of the World Health Organization, emphasized the importance of ensuring public health protocols do not exclude refugees. 'It is vital for all countries to reduce barriers that prevent refugees and migrants from obtaining health care, and to include them in national health policies', he pleaded (WHO, 2020). Instead of banning refugees from entering, countries should have had effective screening and protective measures against communicable diseases. However, despite these calls for compassion, in March 2020, Canada closed its international borders to non-Canadians (Armenski et al., 2021), disregarding pleas from international human rights organizations. Alex Neve, then Secretary-General of Amnesty International Canada, argued vehemently that Canadian borders must always remain open to those seeking protection:

> Canada's decision is out of step with public health measures designed to curb the spread of COVID-19 and runs counter to our international legal obligations. From moral, public health and legal perspectives, closing the border to refugee claimants is wrong. Turning refugee claimants away – including as a result of the decision to shut down the Canada/US border – exposes refugees, who face increased hardship, danger and ostracization worldwide related to this pandemic, to serious human rights violations, including inhumane immigration detention conditions and the risk of refoulement to torture and other human rights abuses. (CCR et al., 2020)

Refugees faced a heightened risk of contracting the COVID-19 virus and experienced worsened health outcomes due to inadequate living conditions, often characterized by overcrowded and unsanitary spaces (Fouad et al., 2021). Nagi et al. (2021) describe how the rates of transmission of the virus were influenced by the congested physical environment of refugees, which frequently lacked sufficient access to clean water, soap, personal protective equipment like masks and gloves, and medicine. The pandemic led to widespread economic disruptions globally, and Syria was no exception. The struggling economy faced further challenges due to public lockdowns and decreased trade. The COVID-19 pandemic also inflicted profound strains on Syria's already fragile healthcare system, with limited hospital beds, disrupted access to medicine and hospital equipment, and many healthcare workers impacted by the fatal virus (UNHCR, 2020).

Meanwhile, in Canada, the impact of the pandemic cannot be overstated. As of 18 January, 2022, the Canadian government reported approximately 2.82 million active COVID-19 cases and 32,220 deaths (Government of Canada, 2022c). In Canada, the response to the pandemic was marred by disorganization and inconsistency. Bryant et al. (2020) shed light on the multifaceted nature of COVID-19's impact on the Canadian population. They argued that the effects were not uniform but were rather racialized, gendered, and affected by socioeconomic class. Indeed, marginalized communities, including newcomer and racialized communities, bore a disproportionate burden of the pandemic's consequences, facing higher infection rates, limited access to healthcare services, and exacerbated economic hardships due in part to the closures of public schools and other public spaces such as libraries and recreational facilities. In a press conference about the provincial restrictions, Ontario's premier Doug Ford stated: 'This virus could hit any one of you or your loved ones because this virus doesn't discriminate. It doesn't care about your race, religion, or creed. It doesn't care about your age. Anyone and everyone is at risk' (Maclean's, 2020).

While the phrase 'the virus does not discriminate' was echoed through mainstream Canadian media channels and political platforms, the data suggest that society, in fact, does discriminate who the virus impacts and to what extent. COVID-19 disproportionately affected equity-seeking communities, including communities of colour, persons with disabilities, and populations residing in confined communal spaces such as shelters and prisons. Refugees in Canada encountered explicit barriers to financial and social support, as well as access to healthcare, education, and social services, during the pandemic (Edmonds and Flahalt, 2021). Canada's response to the pandemic exposed deep-rooted societal issues. The liberal-welfare state model, while praised for its inclusivity and social safety nets, revealed its weaknesses in the face of a crisis of this magnitude. The pandemic starkly illuminated existing inequalities and shortcomings in Canada's healthcare, social, and economic systems, demanding immediate reform and more significant support for those most affected. For example,

Public Health Ontario's epidemiological summary revealed that the virus most severely impacted Ontario's ethnically and culturally diverse neighbourhoods, with higher rates of transmission and severe outcomes such as hospitalizations and deaths (Public Health Ontario, 2021).

Disability defined

While the terms 'disability' and 'disabled' have been used interchangeably to describe one's experiences related to health conditions, impairments, environmental exclusion and identity related to those experiences, my focus lies particularly on the concept of disablement as a dynamic process, as elucidated by Jampel (2018) and Gorman (2018). This process involves the categorization of individuals as disabled, shaped by both the social construction and social production of becoming and being disabled. Gorman explores anticolonial approaches to disability arts, emphasizing disablement's fluidity across social, political, and economic contexts. In this perspective, disablement transcends linear or static definitions; it traverses boundaries, evolves over time, and fluctuates within different social frameworks. This understanding diverges from disability as a static identity historically framed within a biomedical context, as further explored in Chapter Four.

While interacting with participants, I utilized the term 'disabled' in alignment with the perspective that disablement arises from systemic oppressive practices that perpetuate and reinforce disability (Shakespeare, 2010). This viewpoint recognizes the systemic barriers and societal forces that shape an individual's disability experiences. However, it is crucial to acknowledge the diverse language preferences people use to describe their own disability experiences. During the interviews, I encountered various preferences among participants regarding the terminology they chose to use. Some referred to their children as having special needs, while others described their medical condition as their disability. I made a conscious effort to refrain from imposing my own understanding of politically correct terminology prevalent in the Global North, especially considering that what is considered politically correct in Canada may not be so in other parts of the world.

I have observed many instances where healthcare professionals and social activists correct the language families used to describe their children's behaviours or conditions. For example, in a meeting I attended at a paediatric disability agency, the disability rights advocate corrected a parent who referred to their child's condition as 'a special gift' by responding that disabled persons are not special and that deeming them as such was derogatory. The parent explained, 'But my child is a gift from God, and his condition is a test for us as parents'. The parent's belief that their child was exceptional in the eyes of God was a personal conviction and correcting them involved imposing the activist's perspective as authoritative, a dynamic often observed in settler-colonial contexts.

Moreover, it is essential to acknowledge that words can vary in translation across languages, carrying different connotations and nuances. During the interviews, the Arabic words frequently used to describe disability were translated into impairment or obstruction. For many participants, this term resonated as the most fitting description of their child's condition, integral to their narrative. Some participants reported their child never identifying as disabled before coming to Canada. Instead, they described experiences of being excluded from schools and community spaces due to their unique needs in their home country and local host country. When they came to Canada, they heard diagnostic terms such as 'autism spectrum disorder', 'cerebral palsy' and 'global developmental delay' for the first time, and these terms became a marker of their children's identities. For other participants, their child's disabled identity gave them leverage to come to Canada on humanitarian grounds.

However, once in Canada, the promise of a welcoming, inclusive society quickly collided with the reality that disabled individuals often face exclusion from essential health and social services. While Canada is championed as a country leading in universal healthcare, the reality is that disabled persons are frequently left out of essential health and social services. The rallying cry of the Disability Rights Movement, 'Nothing about us without us', remains as urgent today as it did historically (Charlton, 2000). I urge readers to think about how 'us' is defined. Does it include disabled refugees? Ableist policies that perpetuate the segregation of disabled individuals have far-reaching consequences, affecting various aspects of social life, including education, employment, and access to social services (Rioux and Prince, 2002). In 2000, the Department of Citizenship and Immigration took a significant step by exempting Convention refugees (those who are fleeing persecution) and their dependents from the excessive demand clause: 'It is inconsistent for Canada to accept that a Convention refugee overseas is in need of protection but treat them as inadmissible because they would cause excessive demands on health services' (Government of Canada, 2022b). This recognition was particularly crucial for disabled refugees, whose healthcare needs were unfairly stigmatized and deemed burdensome (CCD, 2012). This discrepancy between Canada's professed commitment to refugee rights and its treatment of disabled refugees underscores a fundamental hypocrisy in the nation's approach to refuge, and universal healthcare for all. This theme will be further explored in Chapter Four, where theoretical underpinnings will shed light on the complexities of disablement and displacement.

In Canada today, the exclusion of disabled individuals permeates every facet of social life. Not only are disabled persons subjected to state-sanctioned services and prevailing cultural norms dictating their personal, social, and professional lives, but they are also systematically excluded from decision-making processes at local, provincial, and federal levels. As underscored by Kayess and French (2008), this exclusion from policymaking deprives disabled persons of the opportunity to contribute their perspectives and lived experiences. Consequently, it perpetuates harmful and oppressive ableist practices that continually shape societal norms and structures (Dossa, 2009; Ingstad and Whyte, 2007).

CHAPTER 2
The power of stories

Human stories have the profound ability to communicate powerful messages that transcend time and space, forging transnational connections between families and communities. Stories are more than entertainment or a medium for communication; they serve as vessels for preserving ideas and revealing cathartic truths about ourselves, our families, our cultures, and our worldviews. Through storytelling, we illuminate how our lives intersect with the broader global landscape, transcending transnational borders (Dossa, 2009). The Palestinian poet Mourid Barghouti encapsulates this sentiment, asserting, '[i]f you want to dispossess a people, the simplest way to do it is to tell their story and start with "secondly"' (Adichie, 2009). Barghouti emphasizes how we can oppress storytellers by reducing their stories to a lesser status, thereby disempowering them. Historically, dominant groups have appropriated the narrative voice, particularly of vulnerable and oppressed communities (Dossa, 2013). By telling a story about a group of people enough times, it becomes widely accepted. First-person narratives have the power to inform, educate, dispel misconceptions, and challenge existing policies and practices (Atkinson, 1998). Narrative research allows individuals to reclaim their stories by beginning with 'firstly', sharing not just their versions of events but their truths.

It is within this context that I have sought to capture stories of disabled refugees that have long been overlooked. Disability and migration scholars have largely neglected the unique and often marginalized experiences of disabled refugees, whose voices are frequently silenced in both academic and public discourse (Mirza, 2011; Crock et al., 2012; Pisani & Grech, 2015). Dawson (2019) highlights the significant gap in reliable data on disabled migrants and refugees, noting that the United Nations Department of Economic and Social Affairs (UNDESA) lacks comprehensive statistics on the social, environmental, and economic barriers faced by these individuals, as well as the trauma, abuse, or persecution they endure. Recent studies on Syrian refugees in Canada, for example, have largely concentrated on healthcare needs (Pottie et al., 2016), school integration (Massfeller and Hamm, 2019), the private sponsorship program (Hyndman et al., 2017; Hynie, 2018), and housing accessibility (Oudshoorn et al., 2020). However, these studies have not explored the deeper narratives of disablement and displacement. As a result, the stories of disabled refugees remain under-represented.

The danger of the single story

Chimamanda Ngozi Adichie, acclaimed novelist and storyteller, shares the danger of embracing a singular narrative and how it leads to critical misunderstanding (Adichie, 2009). Reflecting on her upbringing, Adichie recounts how she grew up reading only American and British books. As a child, she illustrated characters who did not resemble her when she wrote stories or drew pictures. They had white skin, blonde hair, and blue eyes. They wore button-down shirts and ironed pleated pants and spoke perfect English. Adichie (2009) describes how vulnerable humans are in the face of a single story that is created by showing 'a people as one thing, as only one thing, over and over again, and that is what they become'. Dominant narratives influence policies and practices by reiterating this single story, and it is only that one story that becomes the widely accepted truth.

Dominant narratives storm our daily lives, saturating newspapers and history books, echoing continually on radio waves and television screens, and presenting a singular perspective on intricate and diverse stories. They shape classroom lessons and influence ideas perpetuated in literature, music, film, art (Razack, 1998), and social media. Dominant cultural narratives are 'systems of representation' (Hasford, 2016, p. 159). They have specific heroes and villains and are void of critical reflection and discourse. Dominant colonial and settler-colonial narratives have been regurgitated through the retelling of a single story of Global North whiteness, white supremacy and power, and the erasure of real-life histories and narratives of those who are racialized, those from the Global South, and those who have been expelled to the Global North.

Real-life stories can be erased by carefully changing the narrative by the listener or observer, rewriting a false record, or not providing space for non-dominant stories to exist (Mothoagae, 2018). In order for the storytellers to tell their truths and be heard, they needed a safe space to share real experiences and oppressions without judgement. As Dr Muna Saleh (2017, p. 41) expresses, in describing her decision to wear hijab in a predominantly white environment, '[a]lthough the stories shift depending upon the beholder, I often feel the weight of each beholder's single story (Adichie, 2009) of who/what I am and who/what I should be like in their stories of a woman who wears hijab'.

Dominant stories influence public perception. A glaring illustration of this occurred with the portrayal of the 2021 London, Ontario, terrorist attacker by mainstream media. Despite the brutal murder of a Muslim family in broad daylight, the image presented on news outlets depicted the perpetrator smiling in a track-and-field picture (Taccone, 2021). The positive image rewrites the story of a domestic terrorist who believed in and acted upon a white supremacy ideology into that of an average young aspiring athlete who committed a heinous act yet is naturally incapable of committing such a heinous attack in the eyes of the public. Dominant narratives oppress non-dominant stories by taking them over while obscuring the very means that produced them (Ryu and Tuvilla, 2018). These stories tell us what and who is important in society, who has power, and who can be cast aside (Dossa, 2008). They are not passive tales that can be easily dismissed; they shape global economic, social, and political movements, offering insight into how society wrestles with its most pressing challenges.

The power of dominant stories is illustrated in the emotional story of Sarah and Yusra Mardini. Yusra, a Syrian refugee who won her heat in the 100-meter butterfly swimming race at the Rio Olympics representing the refugee team, made international headlines in 2022 when her story became widely known with the release of the Netflix movie *The Swimmers*. The Mardini sisters fled Syria on a small dinghy across the Aegean Sea. Shortly after they escaped Syria, their boat's engine failed, and the two sisters risked their lives by swimming for hours in the dark and open freezing water, pushing the boat and saving the others on board. While the Mardini sisters were hailed as heroes, risking their lives to save others, Sarah Mardini's story was received quite differently than her sister Yusra's. After escaping the war, Sarah continued to advocate for and rescue forcibly displaced persons fleeing Syria while going to Greece on boats like the one Sarah used, the same way she escaped Syria. Greek authorities arrested Sarah for assisting asylum seekers on charges of smuggling, fraud and espionage. She spent over a hundred days in prison before having the baseless charges against her completely dropped (Schack and Witcher, 2021). Reflecting on Sarah's story prompts the following question: how could a young woman who risked everything to save the lives of innocent civilians seeking asylum be punished and imprisoned? How can a story change so rapidly, turning the very act that once made her a hero into a criminal. While the heroic story of the Mardini sisters is widely known through the Netflix movie, Sarah's imprisonment adds a complex layer to the dominant narrative surrounding asylum seekers, reinforcing dangerous tropes.

The dominant narrative: welcoming refugees in Canada

In recent decades, the global demand for refuge among forcibly displaced persons has surged dramatically, while the willingness of countries—particularly in the Global North—to offer protection has significantly declined (Bose, 2020). The political reactions from the Global North to the Syrian refugee crisis, in particular, have sparked ongoing debates about the international right to seek asylum, even for those considered especially vulnerable, such as disabled persons (Bose, 2020). The dominant narratives around disabled Syrian refugees exist within a realm of ableist, xenophobic, and Islamophobic ideas. These narratives reiterate disturbing portrayals of refugees as terrorists, victims, criminals, and invaders (Baker and McEnery, 2005) – these narratives also influence who comes to Canada as refugees and how they are perceived and treated. Razack (1998) argues that the stories of refugees found in dominant cultural narratives often overlook the colonial legacy imposed on the Global South by the Global North. In a similar vein, Meekosha (2008, p. 2) eloquently states, '[d]isability studies coming out of the global north assumes the south', suggesting that disability frameworks developed in the Global North fail to account for the experiences of disabled persons in the Global South.

The historical legacy of exclusion is also evident in Canada's own immigration policies. Although portrayed as a welcoming refuge for displaced persons, this image stands in stark contrast to its historically exclusionary immigration policies. While refugee advocates and international humanitarian organizations frame Canada's resettlement efforts as acts of protection and compassion, a closer examination reveals a more complex history. Historically, refugee protection in Canada has been driven by economic interests rather than humanitarian concerns (Heibert, 2016), which systematically discriminates against undesirable immigrants. One of the most notable examples of this exclusionary history is the tragic 1914 incident involving the *Komagata Maru*, a ship carrying 376 racialized immigrants who were denied entry to Vancouver, British Columbia. Kazimi (2012) argues this event exposes Canada's historically racist immigration system, which has traditionally excluded those who do not conform to the idealized image of the desirable immigrant: middle-class, white, and non-disabled settlers. Furthermore, the experiences and processes of becoming a refugee are influenced and shaped by intersecting factors such as ethnicity, gender, and race. In 2001, the Immigration and Refugee Protection Act (IRPA) introduced some changes to Canada's immigration and refugee policies, including a policy that made it feasible for the increased resettlement of refugees with lower literacy rates and education levels, resulting in an increasing number of refugees from countries in the Global South (Hyndman, 2011). This shift appears to reflect a more inclusive approach to refugee resettlement. The widespread national narrative depicting Canada as welcoming refugees with open arms gained prominence over the years, particularly during the political debates of 2015 and 2016 in Canada and the United States. As Bose (2020, p. 3) suggests:

> In Canada, the momentum to resettle a large number of Syrian refugees became enmeshed in the 2015 Canadian general election, with the victorious Liberal Party headed by Justin Trudeau making the acceptance of Syrians a central part of its election platform. In the US, the opposite was true, with Donald Trump making the rejection of Syrians an important part of his winning presidential campaign in 2016. The outcomes of these national elections and the centrality of a particular refugee crisis to each is not simply about the significance of domestic interests vis-à-vis refugee policies.

Canada developed a global image as a saviour for Syrian refugees, juxtaposed against the United States' portrayal of a white nationalist position that rejects them as foreigners. A 2017 CNN report summarizes the opposing reactions to the Syrian refugee crisis with the headline: 'Trump halts refugee program; Trudeau tweets they are welcome in Canada' (Ahmed, 2017). The US media portrayal of Syrian refugees was immediately framed within the context of 9/11 and the 'war on terror' (Rettberg and Gajjala, 2015). On 27 January 2017, Donald Trump issued an official executive order titled 'Protecting the Nation from Foreign Terrorist Entry into the United States' (White House Press Secretary, 2017). This direct federal register order linked the 11 September 2001 attacks to potential incoming terrorists. Terms within the order, such as 'foreign-born' and 'would-be terrorists', underscored its intentions. The proclamation reads: 'deteriorating conditions in certain countries due to war, strife, disaster, and civil unrest increase the likelihood that terrorists will use any means possible to enter the United States' (ibid., p. 2).

The executive order limited travel and settlement for individuals from Muslim-majority countries, including Syria (Liptak and Shear, 2018; Tanfani, 2016). Concurrently, US media outlets depicted arriving refugees with images portraying dishevelled bearded, angry men, explicitly associating terms such as thieves, terrorists, and invaders with them. These images perpetuate narratives portraying Syrian men not only as savage but also as cowards who could not endure hardships in their own country or as freeloaders exploiting the resources of the country willing to accept them (Rettberg and Gajjala, 2015).

Furthermore, the absence of families in media portrayals of Syrian refugees fuels the perception that it is only the men who are entering North America. It reaffirms the orientalist notion that Muslim women are abandoned in their home country and require rescuing (ibid., 2015). The 2016 election of Donald Trump shifted the political conversation from the traditional speaking podium to a transnational unstructured social media platform. Trump's use of Twitter and Facebook was unprecedented for a president (Stolee and Caton, 2018). The 45th president targeted many marginalized populations over social media, including Muslims, disabled persons, and particularly Syrian refugees (Scribner, 2017). His comments reduced Syrian refugees to dangerous and worthless people. In one tweet, he wrote, 'Refugees from Syria are now pouring into our great country. Who knows who they are – some could be ISIS?' (Kruglanski et al., 2019). American politicians, academics, and professionals echoed the social media hashtag #RefugeesNOTWelcome.

Several US governors, including then-Governor Mike Pence, opposed the resettlement of Syrian refugees in their states (Zong and Batalova, 2017). Pence specifically banned Syrian refugees from settling in Indiana, citing concerns for the safety and security of his constituents (Gowayed, 2020). This bold stance reflects the permeation of Islamophobic and xenophobic rhetoric into government policies and practices. A 2016 submission by the Center for Migration Studies titled 'How robust refugee protection policies can strengthen human and national security' further emphasizes the impact of such rhetoric on government policy: 'Refugees and other forcibly displaced persons have fled violence, persecution, and other untenable situations. The overwhelming majority seeks a level of protection and security to which they are legally entitled. At the same time, large-scale refugee and migrant streams include persons with a mix of motives (some dangerous) and aspirations (some illiberal)' (Kerwin, 2016, p. 84).

The messaging north of the Canadian border took a different tone. In January 2017, Prime Minister Justin Trudeau tweeted: 'To those fleeing persecution, terror and war, Canadians will welcome you, regardless of your faith. Diversity is our strength #WelcomeToCanada' (Hughes, 2019). This announcement of welcome framed Canada as a country willing to accept displaced persons fleeing persecution regardless of race, ethnicity, and religion, a refreshing message for racialized Muslims who have been framed as a security threat to society in the post-9/11 era. While the difference between Canadian and American media portrayals of Syrian refugees is stark, Canadian media outlets have also shaped a precarious narrative of Syrian refugees. A February 2016 CBC article titled 'How Syrian refugees arriving in Canada became "extras" in their own stories' sums up the homogonous narrative Canadians have embraced regarding Syrian refugees. This narrative depicts Canada as a global leader accepting displaced persons that other countries will not accept (Tyyska et al., 2018). However, the dominant focus on Canada's acceptance of refugees often overshadows the quality-of-life refugees face once they arrive and settle. Kamal Al-Solaylee, a Canadian journalist and professor, expresses reservations about the portrayal of this welcome:

> Al-Solaylee says he understands why stories about acts of kindness and refugees' first visits to Tim Hortons resonate with journalists and their audiences. However, he worries feel-good stories are 'suck[ing] the oxygen' out of critical

stories about what life in Canada is like for immigrants and refugees after the welcome. The truth is a lot of these immigrants will struggle, initially and probably for a long time. They will not be able to find jobs that call on their qualifications or experience. They will end up doing the kind of work that Canadians no longer want to do. (CBC Radio, 2016)

Those accepted in Canada are often perceived as 'fortunate' and expected to express their gratitude for the country's protection. Being 'accepted' as a refugee is portrayed as a privilege rather than a fundamental human right. This framing of acceptance means the mistreatment of refugees as Canadian newcomers can go without notice. Political leaders and media outlets highlight stories of resilient refugees who have succeeded socially and economically, such as Tareq Hadhad, a Syrian refugee who founded Peace by Chocolate. Prime Minister Justin Trudeau highlighted Hadhad's work at the United Nations Leaders' Summit on Refugees as an example of the opportunities Canada affords newcomers (Bisset, 2016). Hadhad, in an interview on *This Hour Has 22 Minutes*, expresses his love and admiration for Canadians and the favourable treatment he received upon arrival. There is no doubt that real stories of entrepreneurial and financial success exist, but it is essential to recognize that this is not the reality for the majority of newcomers; the 'rags-to-riches' story of refugees in Canada is rare.

The portrayal of acceptance as a privilege instead of a human right contributes to the absence of critical attention to the struggles and injustices that refugees face upon their arrival and throughout their journey of belonging to Canadian society. The narrative that refugees should feel grateful can overshadow the systemic challenges they encounter, such as difficulties in finding meaningful employment, accessing adequate education, and obtaining fair healthcare. This narrative also conceals the fact that refugees have a right to seek asylum under international laws, specifically the 1951 Refugee Convention, and have the right to be treated with dignity and respect (UNHCR, 2024b). While success stories like that of Tareq Hadhad are inspiring and demonstrate the potential of refugees to contribute positively to their new communities, they are only part of the picture. Many refugees continue to face significant barriers, including language obstacles, cultural adjustments, and discrimination. Focusing solely on outlier narratives like Hadhad's can minimize the need for systemic changes and the importance of providing comprehensive support to all refugees. It is crucial to balance the success stories with a realistic portrayal of the challenges faced by Syrian refugees, to ensure that their needs are adequately addressed, and their fundamental rights are protected.

It is also essential to note that not all Canadians support refugees coming to Canada, and not all refugees feel welcome. The welcome narrative often gives way to a narrative of imposed gratitude, a theme that emerged from the participants' stories in Chapter Five. Migrants and refugees have increasingly been described as financial burdens to taxpayers and provincial and federal governments. Media headlines, such as 'No space in Windsor's temporary shelters for Toronto refugees' (CBC News, 2018), depict refugees as manipulating social welfare resources and encroaching on spaces reserved for 'true' Canadians, assumingly white Canadians, not Indigenous peoples. The *Toronto Sun*, amongst other news outlets, frequently highlighted how Canadians would have to pay for the lives of refugees with their tax dollars, framing the acceptance of refugees in terms of the public's financial burden (Levy, 2019). This dominant narrative trickles down into policies that impact the real lives of refugees. While Canada maintains an outward image of appreciating the diversity and cultural enrichment refugees bring to the country, shifts in exclusive policies and practices suggest a different reality (Olsen et al., 2016).

An example of exclusionary policies and subsequent discriminatory practices is the Interim Federal Health Program (IFHP) changes in 2012 that reduced primary healthcare for refugees. The new programme covered only healthcare services deemed essential and acute, which disproportionately affected disabled refugees in Canada who may require prescription medications, adaptive equipment and medical devices, and numerous healthcare consultations with different clinicians. These changes exemplify how prevailing cultural narratives can shape federal policies (Olsen et al., 2016). Although the IFHP was reinstated in 2016 (Chen et al., 2018), the drastic changes illustrate the precarious nature of refugee rights in Canada, often subject to the whims of political actors (Bose, 2020). Bose (ibid.) echoes this fragility in a study examining reactions from government officials working with refugees in Canada and the United States. Notably, one officer in the study referenced a proposed federal 'Barbaric Cultural Practices' hotline to call out unusual or violent behaviours of immigrants and refugees (Gravelle, 2018). Critics of the hotline called out the Islamophobic and racist assumptions embedded in such an initiative (Bose, 2020; Boudjikanian, 2021), which underscore the harmful impact of dominant narratives on policies that directly affect the lives and well-being of marginalized communities.

Concerning dominant stories told for or about them, refugee stories can become alternative stories (White and Epston, 1990), overlooked and unrealized (McMahon, 2007). Contrary to the common perception that refugees undergo a process of restarting or rewriting their life stories upon seeking refuge, the reality is quite different. Refugees are actively experiencing their transnational life stories throughout their displacement journey. The narratives shared by the storytellers in this book stand in stark contrast to the dominant narratives that inform policies and practices concerning disabled refugees. These alternative narratives provide a crucial counterpoint, offering insights into the lived realities of individuals whose voices are often marginalized or overlooked. Through my interactions with the storytellers, I gained invaluable insights into their experiences, uncovering aspects of their stories that may have gone unnoticed.

CHAPTER 3
Collecting the stories

Within the dominant narrative, the refugee experience is often misrepresented as a homogenous one – a single story repeated and rephrased to fit the desired social and political framing of those in dominant positions of power and privilege. However, real human stories, and their connectedness to others can only be understood by paying attention to social, political, and economic contexts. As Dossa (2018, p. 25) notes, '[t]o grasp the meaning of the storied content and the multiple ways in which it is expressed, we must pay attention to the larger sociopolitical contexts that suggest the complex ways in which individuals are connected to the world'.

In writing this book, I find myself situated in a time when disregarding the current geopolitical and socioeconomic climate, both locally and globally, would be a blatant disregard for the realities of today. Humanitarian organizations, including those advocating for disability rights, seem increasingly obsolete as they plea for the upholding of international human rights law, push for political stabilization, and call for an end to global violence. Health disparities among racialized and disabled persons have significantly increased due to the myriad of global health issues as the world continues to grapple with the effects of the COVID-19 pandemic, settler colonialism and health-related sanctions on the Global South by powers in the Global North, and the destruction of the planet by multinational corporations and military conflicts.

Racialized communities in Canada continue to endure profound and ongoing harm that is largely overlooked. The discovery of hundreds of Indigenous children's bodies in the grounds of residential schools across Canada has elicited only a faint public outcry (Norris, 2021). Meanwhile, Black Lives Matter protests persist across North American, exposing the systemic and pervasive anti-Black racism that permeates our institutions (Mullings et al., 2016). Islamophobia in Canada has reached unprecedented levels, marked by the 2017 Quebec Mosque shooting that killed six congregants in a mosque and injured five others, and the 2021

London terrorist attack, where a white supremacist deliberately ploughed down a Muslim family in broad daylight because they were perceived as foreigners and invaders (AlJazeera, 2021). I write this book at a time when wearing a hijab, as I do, or a turban prevents individuals from becoming public school teachers or police officers in Quebec due to discriminatory laws that police certain garments and symbols (NCCM, 2021). Furthermore, advocating for the rights of persecuted populations, such as Palestinians, makes one a political target and results in censorship by the very academic institutions that pride themselves on freedom of speech and thought. It is crucial to note that while disabled Syrian refugees may have entered Canada, ignoring the local and global context of systemic discrimination and institutionalized exclusion would be a disgrace to the very humans who trusted me with their stories.

Collecting the stories went beyond the routine steps of interviewing participants, transcribing their interviews, and reviewing and analysing those transcripts. As Elder (2015) aptly notes, the depth and richness of the stories and experiences of disabled refugees often get clouded by clinical protocols and quantitative checklists. These rigid frameworks fail to capture the complexities of their multiple and intersecting identities, daily experiences, and real-life oppressions and make it easier for policymakers, service providers, and educators to ignore the critical intersectional needs of disabled refugees. While interviewing participants and gathering their stories are standard practices in qualitative research, my approach to this process was intentional, purposeful, and deeply significant. I carefully considered the approach I would use to gain an understanding from the participants I spoke with, as it was imperative to collect their stories in the most dignified ways, using a methodology that honoured their time and energy and prioritized their needs above all else. After careful deliberation, narrative inquiry, the study of stories (Andrews et al., 2008), emerged as the ideal approach. This was the most suitable method for capturing the complex web of personal, national, and transnational narratives surrounding displacement and disablement.

As qualitative researchers Clandinin and Connelly (2006) propose, narrative inquiry, which involves studying experiences through storytelling, can shape how we perceive and understand those experiences. Our individual stories are not isolated entities but are intricately woven into personal, social, and institutional narratives (Clandinin et al., 2011; Clandinin and Rosiek, 2007). These narratives of experiences are not static; they are dynamic, evolving through living, telling, retelling, and reliving one's story (Clandinin and Connelly, 2000; Lawlor and Mattingly, 2000). In the intimate space of our conversations, I witnessed first-hand how participants' stories were relived repeatedly. Their tears, smiles, and shrugs served as poignant reminders of the emotional depth and complexity embedded within their narratives. These moments underscored the profound transformative impact of storytelling as a form of self-expression.

Through the act of sharing their stories, participants asserted their agency by claiming and reclaiming ownership of their narratives. Their willingness to convey deeply personal accounts highlights a few key points. First, it underscores the importance of creating safe spaces that honour lived experiences, reaffirming the power of narrative inquiry in eliciting authentic, nuanced accounts of human experiences. Second, by actively and intentionally listening to their stories, I gained deeper insights into the complexities of their lived experiences (Hays and Singh, 2012; Webster and Mertova, 2007). The narrative inquiry methodology was not chosen to recount the stories of the 10 participants; rather, the methodology guided me toward purposefully sharing those stories. As I conversed with the storytellers, I was compelled to reflect on my own responsibility in exploring and sharing the insights I gained. How do I, a Canadian citizen born and raised in Kitchener, Ontario, connect with the story of a refugee who grew up in Damascus, Syria?

Narrative inquiry requires active engagement from the audience or listener (Dossa, 2009). As Dossa (ibid., p. 25) states, '[w]hen readers engage with stories and their various interpretations, new meanings are created that will reverberate in the readers' own local culture and sometimes the dominant culture as well'. Dossa highlights the advocacy potential of storytelling, noting that narratives can bridge gaps between perspectives, fostering empathy and understanding. Narrative research complements traditional scientific inquiry, enhancing, for example, what can be found in data collection through surveys. In this way, storytelling does not just provide insights into individual experiences; it also enriches and deepens broader research findings, offering a more holistic understanding of complex issues.

Limitations to collecting and sharing stories

As with any research methodology, narrative inquiry can be dominated by the researcher holding a position of power (Dossa, 2009). Researchers are not exempt from rewriting stories that perpetuate dominant narratives, and I had to carefully examine my privileges as a researcher throughout the entire research process. As Bochner et al. (2000) argue, we must be critical of who is telling the story, who is sharing it, and the motives behind it. In exploring the narratives of disabled Syrian refugees and their families, I knew these stories had to come directly from the voices of those most impacted—disabled Syrian refugees and their families. As someone who neither identifies as Syrian nor as disabled, it was important that I engaged in critical self-reflection throughout my research journey. According to Frank, A.W. (2000), reflexivity is an essential component of narrative research, helping researchers identify their privilege (Hankivsky, 2012). To ensure I critically reflected on my positionality and privilege in relation to the stories—both individually and collectively—I kept an ongoing journal of reflections. These reflections were crucial in assessing why my study on disablement and displacement held value. Storytelling is not merely about recounting experiences; it demands rigour to uphold a critical yet sincere position and a respectful and dignified approach throughout the entire research journey – from conducting interviews to collecting data to analysing the data and sharing the narratives.

During the data collection phase, several obstacles may have hindered the safe space I aimed to create with the participants. For example, the communication platforms used to connect with the storytellers presented numerous accessibility challenges. With government-imposed COVID-19 restrictions prohibiting in-person interactions with research participants, virtual engagement became necessary. At first, I tried communicating with all participants through the video conferencing software Zoom. However, this was difficult for some participants because they did not have the technology for video conferencing nor could they maintain a stable internet connection, which led to disruptions during our conversations. For example, my session with Marwa was paused several times as the video call became disconnected due to a weak internet connection. At one point, when she reconnected, she began by stating, 'I don't remember where I was, that's okay'. Then she moved on to the next point in her story. Despite my attempts to guide her back to the previous point, it seemed she had mentally transitioned to the next part of her narrative. Similarly, Sarah paused our video call as her child required the only computer they had at home for online learning. Sarah switched from Zoom to a phone call and resumed her story, but talking over the phone was very different as I could no longer observe her facial expressions or gestures.

Using a language interpreter introduced additional barriers, despite the intention to facilitate communication and improve accessibility. On several occasions, the language interpreter interrupted the storyteller during the conversation to translate the information from Arabic to English. While their intention was likely to ensure accurate interpretation, this interruption disrupted the conversational rhythm and potentially prevented participants from completing their thoughts. Additionally, participants may have felt uneasy or frustrated waiting for me to obtain the information in English from the interpreter, potentially altering the course of our discussions.

Stories unveiled amidst chaos

My first interview took place on 6 January 2021. It was a day marked by chaos. It was the day white supremacists stormed the US Capitol building in broad daylight (Willingham, 2021). As I observed the attack unfolding on television in disbelief, witnessing the assault of police officers and damage of government property, it felt like a bold display of the power and privilege of white supremacists for all to witness. I could not shake the question of whether others saw what I saw – a day of turmoil that will unfold in North American history within a dominant narrative framing the perpetrators as disobedient but civil. The 45th President of the United States went as far as defending the actions of what he labelled as lawful protestors, refraining from categorizing them as criminals or terrorists (ibid.). Instead of the brute police force we often see with brown and black protestors, there was a surprising delicacy in how these white insurrectionists were treated.

During that first interview on 6 January 2021, I was taken aback to hear Hassan's story. He shared how the police came to his home recently to deliver a final eviction notice that cited noise complaints.

Hassan explained how his children are nonverbal and make vocalizations to express themselves. Hassan recounted how his white neighbours frequently called the police over the noise, subjecting his family to relentless harassment and derogatory remarks, such as urging them to 'go back where they came from' – a phrase that resonated painfully with me and one that I am sure many racialized persons are subjected to. With tears in his eyes, Hassan revealed his fear of law enforcement and his bewilderment at the cruelty directed towards his children, particularly as refugees to Canada with disabled children. He pleaded with his landlord not to call the police, sharing how he could not prevent his children from making noise. Hassan recounted the hostility and insensitivity exhibited by the police during their visits and drew a comparison between the police in Canada and the police he encountered during the security checkpoints when seeking asylum in Egypt. He was subjected to interrogations about his occupation and immigration status and was continuously expected to provide explanations of his children's behaviours – then and now. Despite his earnest attempts to explain, police officers remained unsympathetic towards his children's conditions. Hassan and I never discussed the irony of that day, but I spent hours reflecting on his story after I hung up, wondering whether he felt the same hypocrisy I did.

CHAPTER 4
Theoretical underpinnings

While existing frameworks found in critical migration studies and critical disability studies have largely ignored the disabled refugee (Reilly, 2010; Pisani, 2012; Burns, 2017), the combination of theoretical frameworks presented in this chapter will provide a vital perspective to examine the issues that impact disabled Syrian refugees within both a local and transnational context. Concepts of citizenship, otherness, and intersectionality inform this narrative study of disablement and displacement. It is situated within a critical paradigm of transnational disablement, which I will elaborate further in the coming sections.

Although my research does not explicitly explore a historically rooted materialist perspective, the core tenets of the theory that underlie exclusionary immigration and disability policy can be expressed in terms of economic undesirability. Returning to the question posed in Chapter One by Butler (1993) – why do only some bodies matter? – Erevelles (2011) urges us to question the historical material conditions that determine why certain bodies are valued more than others. Those bodies, for example, that are located at the intersections of race, disability, and gender are socially and economically determined as inferior by the very establishments devised to safeguard them. Fundamental human rights, such as those discussed by the participants, are linked with '[e]conomic conditions that sustain the unequal social relations of class. These unjust economic arrangements are obscured by the development of discourses of morality that justify those who are denied this right by categorizing them as "the undeserving"' (Erevelles, 2002, p. 15).

Models of disability

To begin this theoretical analysis, I explore the multifaceted relationship between disablement and displacement by examining both traditional and contemporary models of disability. The prevailing discourse on disability in the Global North, situated within settler colonialism and whiteness, is primarily influenced by the biomedical model of disability. This model perpetuates the notion that there is a singular, ideal way to look, communicate, move, learn, and exist. It posits non-disabled as natural, whereas differences in appearance, communication, movement, and behaviour that result from a condition, illness, or impairment are viewed as unfit, unnatural, and undesirable.

The biomedical model frames disability as rooted in an individual's pathology (Smart, 2005) and focuses on the impairment of the body and the treatments and cures of ailments that tarnish the body (Schur et al., 2013). In this regard, the biomedical model equates disability to a problem that requires changing or fixing (Oliver, 2004). A vital feature of the rhetoric of this model of disability is the assertion that being non-disabled is normal and being disabled is abnormal. Such classification is catastrophic because every aspect of a disabled person's life becomes regulated to fit into the 'typical' or 'normal' archetype. The biomedical model largely ignores one's culture, physical and social environment (Oliver and Barnes, 2012), geopolitical context, and personal narrative and history. It overlooks critical social determinants of health and disability that impact the everyday lives of disabled refugees.

The social model of disability shifts the focus away from curing, preventing, or rehabilitating disability, and instead examines the ableist policies and practices that exclude and harm disabled individuals (ibid.). By challenging social barriers, the model rejects the idea that disability is solely an individual problem (Rolston, 2014; Morris, 2001). Building on the social model, Dawson (2019) introduces the 'Social Model of Refugeeness,' a framework that advocates for a shift in societal perceptions of dependence among refugees. Dawson emphasizes how authentic representations of disabled refugees offer valuable insights into the refugee experience, particularly during moments of displacement. This framework explores the historical context that creates a disabling environment for the refugee, examines how refugee agency is constrained, and highlights the acts of resistance refugees employ in response to these challenges.

While the social model of disability emphasizes social, economic, and political factors surrounding disablement, it fails to address systemic barriers affecting specific disabled populations (Frank, G., 2000), such as disabled refugees. Furthermore, it recognizes disability within a Global North context and ignores intersectional factors of experience (Rose, 2020) and oppression. The social model's effectiveness in addressing the diverse experiences of disabled individuals remains a subject of debate within critical disability discourse as it brushes over the narratives and lived realities of disabled persons. For example, it overlooks how global systems of oppression—such as armed conflict, occupation, settler colonialism, and apartheid—contribute to disablement.

The human rights model of disability underscores human diversity and embraces disability as one of several layers of human identity (Rioux et al., 2011). Taking a social justice approach, it urges those in positions of authority to assume a moral position, a seeming improvement to the social model of disability. The human rights approach underscores the need for legislation and public policies that support the full involvement of all persons, regardless of sociopolitical affiliation, economic status, or sociocultural factors (Kayess and French, 2008). Within this framework, no life is deemed inferior to another based on differences in physical, mental, cognitive, or sensory abilities, illnesses, or impairments. Such categorizations would violate principles of equality and social justice (Rioux and Carbert, 2003). Human rights discourse has played a key role in determining who is considered worthy of rights and who is not. This is shaped by influential and powerful actors who decide which freedoms are deemed deserving (Kazemi, 2019). Amongst the undeserving or under-deserving are disabled refugees. The claim that all humans have human rights by virtue of being human is an ideological stance that must account for the social, economic, and political means by which we obtain our rights. Furthermore, discussions about morality often conceal explicit and implicit human rights violations. These violations are rarely acknowledged as systemic and institutionalized, even within human rights discourse, and are rooted in broader structures of oppression. As Farmer (2005) argues, these rights violations are not accidental nor are they isolated incidents, but manifestations of deeper power imbalances connected with economic and social conditions that determine whose rights will be protected and upheld and whose will be ignored and abused.

The United Nations Convention on the Rights of Persons with Disabilities (CRPD) and its optional protocol were formed in response to international human rights instruments' exclusion of disability rights (Degener, 2016). The CRPD marked a pivotal milestone in upholding the rights of persons with disabilities by formalizing fundamental and practical concerns raised by the disability community (Kayess and French, 2008), including a call to end the dehumanizing practices of institutionalizing disabled persons (Karsay and Lewis, 2012). The CRPD was the first international human rights instrument to acknowledge disabled persons as human rights holders and recognize that illness, impairment, or disability could not be used as justification for denying human rights (Crock et al., 2017; Degener, 2016).

The CRPD was not designed to create or implement new rights but to realize and apply existing rights to persons with disabilities, thereby moving disabled persons into the deserving-of-rights category. Disabled persons include both citizens and non-citizens, such as displaced persons (Crock et al., 2017). The CRPD had a tremendous global impact on how societies view disabled persons and the need to improve their overall social and economic conditions (Kayess and French, 2008). It clarified the right of disabled persons to have and exercise legal capacity and significantly influenced international human rights law and disability studies (Degener, 2016). For example, Article 11 of the CRPD, 'Situations of Risk and Humanitarian Emergencies', highlights that disabled persons, including displaced disabled persons, must have their human rights protected. However, critics of Article 11 argue that the CRPD should apply only to citizens of a given state, especially since some countries increasingly have refugees crossing into their borders (Crock et al., 2017). In 2013, with the outcry of leaders in the Global North about the perceived social and economic strain Syrian refugees were placing on Global North countries, the CRPD reiterated its obligation to apply the Convention to all individuals, regardless of nationality or citizenship status: 'Syria is a State Party to the Convention on the Rights of Persons with Disabilities. Article 11 of the Convention states:

> Parties shall take, in accordance with their obligations under international law, including international humanitarian law and international human rights law, all necessary measures to ensure the protection and safety of persons with disabilities in situations of risk, including situations of armed conflict, humanitarian emergencies and the occurrence of natural disasters (United Nations, 2006).

While the CRPD has made significant strides in highlighting the concerns of disabled persons globally, and the need for countries to realize disabled persons' rights, it is essential to recognize that the CRPD was developed within a historical framework of disability rights activism, grounded in whiteness. This framework has ignored the historical and material contexts in which disability is situated (Gorman, 2016). Although universal human rights instruments such as the CRPD have wielded considerable influence over international human rights discourse (Meekosha and Soldatic, 2011), the human rights paradigm, like the biomedical and social models, has been developed in the Global North within a Eurocentric colonial-settler context where Indigenous populations have been displaced and replaced by settler populations (Veracini, 2015), which is a point ignored in many disability discourses.

Furthermore, the CRPD involves a concept of universalism that reiterates disabled persons as a homogenized population (Bickenbach, 2009; WHO, 2015). Countries worldwide may agree to universal human rights principles, but those principles are defined by wealthy and powerful players (Meekosha and Soldatic, 2011; Sen, 2009). This dynamic is evident in the permanent members' veto power at the United Nations Security Council, which allows powerful countries to block or influence international resolutions, including those related to upholding and protecting basic human rights (Iyase and Folarin, 2018) by defining who is worthy of them. As Kazemi (2018, p. 201) writes, 'a "universal" idea of disablement has abysmally failed, because transnational, local, and international advocacy groups do not fight for equality for disabled people in the "third world." Instead, they just fight for their "survival"'. A striking example of this failure in recent history is the United Nations' repeated inability to secure a ceasefire in Gaza, primarily due to the United States exercising its veto power multiple times in 2023 and 2024. Amnesty International's Secretary General, Agnes Callamard, along with other human rights leaders, has condemned the U.S. for using its veto to manipulate the UN Security Council, thereby undermining its credibility and effectiveness in upholding international peace and security (Amnesty International, 2023). This failure to protect the human rights of all individuals—particularly women, children, and people with disabilities—reveals deep flaws within the global human rights system. It underscores the urgent need for collective efforts to address systemic inequalities and entrenched power imbalances, especially those rooted in the Global North that continue to marginalize and oppress communities in the Global South.

Disability rights activists have relied heavily on the CRPD as the gold standard to advocate for the rights of disabled persons. However, the CRPD fails to adequately address transnational claims to justice around disability. This is primarily because the Convention continues to adopt a nation-state perspective (Soldatic, 2013), overlooking the authentic narratives of who becomes disabled, how, when, and why. Additionally it neglects those who have transitioned from one nation-state to another and who may have a different legal status in the various countries they are forced to reside in. For example, Article 18 of the CRPD, 'Liberty of Movement and Nationality', undoubtedly recognizes the rights of disabled persons to move freely between countries, seek asylum, and leave their own country. While Article 18 appears to afford essential rights to disabled displaced persons, it is crucial to note that states are not obligated to ratify the CRPD. Canada ratified the CRPD in 2010 (Government of Canada, 2020b). Australia, on the other hand has ratified the Convention with an interpretative clause allowing exemption from Article 18 (Meekosha and Soldatic, 2011). Such an exemption effectively absolve countries from the obligation to revise discriminatory migration laws and policies that explicitly exclude disabled displaced persons (El-Lahib and Wehbi, 2012; Soldatic and Fiske, 2009).

The CRPD's focus on the modern territorial state leaves little room for pursuing disability justice rights in relation to transnational or international corporations or institutions (Soldatic and Biyanwila, 2006). As states' economic and political power increasingly transcends national borders, multinational corporations exert disproportionate global influence. Consequently, the pursuit of justice and equity within human rights frameworks becomes increasingly complex due to the significant sway these powerful actors hold. Pisani (2012) highlights the paradox of international human rights instruments that fail to protect humans forcibly displaced from their homes. Nation-states prioritize protection of their citizens against perceived threats, controlling their borders and determining who is allowed membership. Unsurprisingly, refugees and asylum seekers are often deemed the perceived threat (Scott and Safdar, 2017). While the language of human rights may generally be framed around all persons' inherent rights, those rights cannot be realized in a disabling system that privileges the rights and freedoms of some persons over others.

Furthermore, while human rights discourse has often been used to champion the rights of individuals, it has also been co-opted to perpetuate violations through settler-colonial and imperialist ideologies (Meekosha & Soldatic, 2011). A notable example lies in the post-9/11 era and the 'war on terror', where human rights rhetoric has predominantly prioritized the security of individuals residing in the Global North (Pisani and Grech, 2015) at the expense of humans in the Global South, reducing the flow of migration from the Global South to the Global North including those escaping persecution.

By framing migration as a privilege rather than a fundamental right, a state's security rhetoric can reshape perceptions of refugees from individuals needing protection to those granted exceptional circumstances (Pisani and Grech, 2015). In Canada, human rights rhetoric has been similarly co-opted to justify discriminatory exclusionary policies such as Bill 21, a Quebec law that disproportionately impacts racialized communities, including new immigrant and refugee communities. Bill 21 bans Canadians who wear religious symbols or garments such as hijabs or turbans from working in public spaces such as police stations, courtrooms, and public schools (National Assembly of Québec, 2019). Bill 21, while framed around the notion of freedom of religion and religious neutrality, instead disproportionally impacts racialized and newcomer communities and limits the social, economic, and political participation of Canadians who adhere to certain faith traditions, such as Sikhism and Islam, and choose to dress a certain way. Research suggests that Muslim women are the most impacted by Bill 21 due to their visible attire (Rukavina, 2022). In this way, human rights language that purports to protect freedoms is used to reinforce systems of exclusion and oppression, particularly for those already marginalized due to race, religion, and immigration status. Bill 21 exemplifies how human rights discourse can reinforce the very inequalities it claims to address. When we highlight non-dominant narratives, we not only draw attention to human rights violations locally and globally, but also call for a critical reevaluation of international human rights instruments that fail to protect all people.

Transnational model of disability

Within disability studies, we have seen the shift in discourse from the biomedical model of disability to the social and human rights models; however, transnational experiences of disability continue to be left out of prominent theoretical disability perspectives. Disability is not solely determined by social circumstances and environmental factors, but is also intricately linked to transnational social, economic, and political contexts. For example, the impacts of armed conflict, structural violence, and physical, psychological, and intergenerational trauma on disabled persons' bodies must be critically examined. Ignoring experiences such as life in a refugee camp, crossing inaccessible checkpoints, and the mass injuries inflicted on tens of thousands of children in the Global South by weapons manufactured in the Global North means neglecting the real transnational experiences of disability. Moreover, the binary distinction between disabled and non-disabled persons inherent in traditional models of disability has often been used to segregate and isolate disabled persons in the Global South as well as migrants in the Global North.

Transnational capitalist material conditions play a significant role in creating and perpetuating circumstances that result in disability, such as deprivation of food, medicine, and daily essentials through ongoing illegal occupations and apartheid in the Global South (Erevelles, 2011). These oppressive systems degrade disabled persons through practices that severely restrict their ability to move, communicate, access services, learn, work, and live freely. While disabled individuals may have legal protections under international or national laws as outlined by the CRPD, these rights often fail to translate into tangible social and economic liberties. This longstanding critique—examining the gap between disability rights advocacy and the realization of those rights—has been reiterated by disability scholars like Vanhala (2010), Jaeger and Bowman (2005), and Davis (1999), among others.

Disability scholars who aim to shift from a biomedical to a social definition of disability often overlook the colonial and capitalist structures that sustain white supremacy within disability discourse. These models fail to address the root causes of *debility* and *disablement* which are critical to understanding disability through a transnational lens. Debility, according to Puar (2017),

[m]arks a state of bodies and populations that have been disabled, disempowered, and incapacitated, but it does so in ways that disavow conventional disability. Debility is a biopolitical condition that works through neglect, violence, and forms of strategic, slow violence that cannot be categorized as straightforwardly 'disabling' in the conventional sense." (Puar, 2017, p. 12).

Debility is intentional; it is a state that makes conditions unliveable, going beyond the traditional notion of disability to examine conditions that result from social, political, and economic barriers imposed on human life. Debility involves the ongoing systematic degradation of the environment and structural violence against specific populations. Puar's, *The Right to Maim* (2017) explores real-life examples of Palestinians becoming disabled due to long-standing targeted violence designed to maim and incapacitate. She draws parallels between disablement experienced by Palestinians in the Global South and black communities in the Global North: 'Ferguson-to-Gaza forums sought to correlate the production of settler space, the vulnerability and degradation of black and brown bodies, the demands for justice through transnational solidarities, and the entangled workings of settler colonialism in the United States and Israel' (ibid., ix).

The comparison between Ferguson and Gaza highlights how interconnected realities of targeted disability and the processes of disablement are within oppressive social, economic, and political environments shaped by settler colonialism. While Puar first wrote about debility in Gaza almost a decade ago, the relevance of her work is even more crucial today as Palestinians experience a genocide, continuing to be ethnically cleansed from their land, mass murdered, forcibly displaced, and deliberately maimed (Albanese, 2024).

Like Puar, Kazemi (2019) emphasizes the social, political, and economic contexts that impact disabled persons by describing the process of disablement, which:

> locates the problem in the violence of global class-relations (capitalism, imperialism, and neo-colonialism), the dialectics of global politics, historical infliction of pain upon the poor and racialized body (e.g., colonialism, slavery, Indigenous genocide, indentured labour, war on terror), exploitative social relations (gendered, raced, and classes), and destruction

of the planet by the ruling bourgeois class causing health issues for every species.

Gorman (2005) prompts us to consider the consequences of overlooking these root causes of disablement which arise from systemic oppressive practices that perpetuate and reinforce disability that create and exacerbate trauma and injury, and perpetuate and amplify social barriers. Gorman (2018) asks: 'What critical representations of disablement have been promoted or sidelined? When does disability emerge as identity, and what assemblages do these identities reference? What happens when we let go of disability identity in representations of war, migration, and sovereignty?' (p. 457). Gorman's questions mark a shift from the traditional focus of disability as an identity that has historically shaped conventional disability models (Kazemi, 2019).

When disabled refugees are resettled in Canada, their transnational experiences of displacement and disablement are frequently disregarded. Instead, they are subjected to lectures about their perceived fortune in being granted human rights and basic privileges in Canada and are pressured to express gratitude as highlighted in Chapter Five. Many participants, while sharing their stories, emphasized how warfare, medical and food sanctions, and forced displacement directly caused their children's disabilities. Why then are critical aspects of debility and disablement often ignored within disability studies?

The 2021 Sienna International Photo of the Year titled 'Hardships of Life', taken by Turkish photographer Mehmet Aslan, portrays Munzir El Nezzel, a Syrian father and his son Mustafa in a Turkish refugee camp. The photograph garnered global attention for its poignant depiction of disability amidst armed conflict. It captures resistance through a transnational disability lens, revealing the parallels of disability experiences across borders and contexts. In this single photograph, we witness the profound impact of military violence on multiple generations within a family. The father, who lost his leg due to a bomb explosion, tenderly holds his child, who was born without arms and legs. The child's disability is directly linked to his mother's exposure to chemical warfare while pregnant, compounded by the inability to seek medical attention due to the sanctions on Syria (Moore, 2022).

Rather than labelling the El Nezzel family members as disabled, we must instead ask critical questions about their disabilities, about *debility* and *disablement*. Their disabilities are not simply biomedical experiences or social constructs. We must ask: How did this young father's leg become amputated? He was walking in a bazaar, buying food for his family. How were the child and mother affected by chemical warfare? Why were they not able to get humanitarian assistance? Why were they not protected? Aslan's photograph challenges us to consider disability within a transnational framework that recognizes the complex intersections of disability and oppressive systems of violence. It forces us to reflect on how disability is intertwined with social, economic, and political challenges that transcend our geographical borders, including transnational human rights violations, and highlights the importance of examining disability experiences within the broader context of global systems and structures of oppression.

Citizenship

Analysing disability within the context of citizenship compels us to challenge the traditional models of disability and associated stereotypes (Prince, 2009). The conceptual framework of citizenship provides a lens through which we can question how individuals are accepted, welcomed, valued, and included in society. Regardless of their citizenship status, disabled individuals often face exclusion and discrimination rooted in ideals perpetuated by the biomedical model, focusing on physical characteristics and disease identification. Disability activists and critical disability scholars use the concept of citizenship to elucidate the social exclusion experienced by disabled persons and advocate for their full participation (Barton, 1993; Hughes, 2014; Prince, 2004; Van Houten and Jacobs, 2005).

Framing disability within the context of citizenship has been instrumental for disability rights movements, as citizenship underscores certain political, social, and economic rights that should be afforded to all. Oliver (1992) argued that citizenship profoundly rejects disability because it entails belonging and inclusion, whereas disabled persons are treated at best as 'second-class citizens' (Barton, 1993; Oliver, 1992). Even when granted legal state citizenship, disabled persons may still encounter social exclusion, being made to feel like non-citizens or partial citizens. While framing disability within the context of citizenship is important, it does not guarantee that disabled persons will receive the same rights as others. Pisani and Grech (2015) argue that when the social model frames disability rights under the banner of citizenship, it assumes citizenship is a given right. However, citizenship literature has largely overlooked the reasons why disabled individuals are prevented from obtaining full citizenship (Rioux and Valentine, 2006). The exclusion of disabled persons from having citizenship rights may result from exclusive social, economic, and legal policies, as well as abusive practices like coerced genetic testing to identify disabilities prenatally.

Historically, citizenship has been a cornerstone of the nation-state concept, defining the rights of individuals within specific geographical borders (Janoski and Gran, 2002). While citizenship has emerged as a central tenet of the liberal state, the boundaries of nation-states have become increasingly blurred due to socioeconomic and political factors such as forced migration and globalization. Consequently, citizenship has evolved to emphasize community membership, aligning more closely with the dominant national culture. Viewing citizenship as membership in a community allows for an analysis of citizenship within the context of prevailing societal norms and values (Yuval-Davis, 1997). However, such membership can also lead to exclusion based on various socially constructed factors, challenging the notion of everyday citizenship for individuals based on their beliefs, country of origin, race, nationality, gender, or ethnicity.

Morris (2005) critiques dominant models of citizenship, which often emphasize self-determination, participation, and especially economic contribution. Perhaps the most controversial point is the latter. Disability scholars criticize the fact that citizenship depends on an individual's ability to contribute to a country's economy. Social welfare systems have often been structured to exclude disabled individuals from the workforce, limiting their social and economic potential. Many disabled persons face chronic exclusion from employment opportunities that prioritize specific skills and abilities over others (Prince, 2009), leading to unemployment, poverty, and reliance on social assistance, which can negatively impact their citizenship status (Arnold, 2004). Disabled persons are perpetually stereotyped as unproductive burdens on the economy (Hahn, 1985) and deemed unworthy of full citizenship (Thobani, 2007). Disabled persons are further viewed as obstructions to neoliberalist and capitalist structures designed to maximize profits (Russell, 2002).

Even prominent political philosophers like John Rawls (1998), known for his work on Justice as fairness in the liberal polity, have been criticized for excluding disabled persons from their definition of citizenship, often employing humanist reasoning (Erevelles, 2011). Humanist ideology prioritizes individual capability regarding competence, rationality, and independence (Garland-Thompson, 1997). Rawls's description implies that a citizen must be a fully 'cooperating member of society' (Rawls, 1998, p. 5). This assumption, rooted in ableist and exclusionary ideals, equates typical work with specific physical and cognitive abilities and traits. Evaluating citizenship based on an individual's capacity to contribute in a particular manner contradicts the notion that citizenship should inherently entail rights, regardless of one's ability to 'give back' to the nation-state (Goodley and Lawthom, 2019).

In Canada, a refugee's path to citizenship is further measured by their competence of 'Canadian-ness', which involves embracing Canadian values and customs, including fluency in Canada's national language(s) and participation in Canadian holidays (Beiser, 2009). Assimilation is necessary to demonstrate allegiance to one's country (Rajaram and Grundy-Warr, 2007). Canada's immigration points system is a crucial example of how dominant cultural norms and narratives dictate what it means to belong, encompassing expected behaviours within society. Membership predominantly favours those who align with normative standards historically defined by traits associated with white, heterosexual, middle-class, and non-disabled men. To conform to neoliberal economic principles, individuals must exhibit a level of capability, competence, rationality, and independence expected in the Global North.

Othering the other

Disabled refugees are repeatedly othered in their relentless and nearly impossible quest for full citizen membership. Disabled refugees are perceived as less capable, less competent, and less able to contribute to society, leading to their devaluation and dehumanization. Global North scholars (including disability and migration scholars) have furthered the discourse on othering, describing the disabled-other and refugee-other similarly, as a misfit archetype, both socially vulnerable and inferior (Fernando and Rinaldi, 2017). Reiterated through historical and present-day processes of colonialism and settler colonialism, systemic othering goes beyond superficial differences or stereotypes, categorizing persons into binary opposites such as citizen versus refugee or non-disabled versus disabled (Bauman, 1991).

Grech (2015, p. 11) suggests, '[c]olonialism not only reframed bodies and disability, but it also impacted how disability was to be engaged with, and on occasion "treated" when met by the colonizer'. In this regard, colonialism rewrites the narratives of disabled persons in the Global South and those who have migrated from the Global South to the Global North. The aim of colonization is to invade a space, exploit resources, cause chaos and disruption, and then return home more powerfully than before. The colonized are left powerless and rely on the colonizers for economic and social support. Grech and Soldatic (2015) suggest that 'the colonizer, in encountering the Other, had to construct that Other in terms of race, culture, body, and spirit'. When the colonized must come into the colonizer's now-territory, they must conform and be able to contribute in a way deemed fit by the newly formed society.

The process of domination within these oppressive systems must be considered when examining disabled refugees' experiences (Grech and Soldatic, 2015; Erevelles, 2011), as they have impacted their lived experiences at every juncture. Resistance to domination must also be examined, as disabled persons rejected being controlled. Erevelles (2014) suggests that the proliferation of disablement has been attributed to colonial and neocolonial rule, which facilitates the establishment of repressive police states aimed at suppressing colonial subjects who resist harmful living conditions imposed upon them.

Drawing on Edward Said's (1978) theory of Orientalism, which explores how colonizers depicted Middle Eastern and Asian cultures as barbaric and inferior, we can examine the power dynamics in this othering process in creating a dominant narrative. Orientalism went beyond stereotypes to create a narrative that dehumanized Eastern cultures while portraying Europeans as modern and civilized. Said criticized Western scholars for biased portrayals that obscured the beauty and diversity of Middle Eastern peoples. For Said (2000,

p. 529), othering is a 'conceptual framework around the notion of us-versus-them [that] is in effect to pretend that the principal consideration is epistemological and natural – our civilization is known and accepted, theirs is different and strange – whereas the framework separating us from them is belligerent, constructed, and situational'.

The process of othering extends beyond geographical boundaries, affecting Arabs and Muslims living in the colonized Global South and refugees residing in the Global North. This pervasive othering paints them as inhumane and uncivilized, leading to discrimination, exclusion, and structural violence. Disabled refugees face an added layer of othering through dominant narratives that uphold a narrow standard of normalcy.

Intersectional oppressions

The othering and exclusion experienced by the participants in this study who shared narratives of transnational disablement were both multifaceted and complex. The storytellers recounted experiences of racism, ableism, xenophobia, and Islamophobia – not as separate issues but as deeply intertwined factors of their lived realities. While disability studies scholars like Ben-Moshe and Magaña (2014), Bailey and Mobley (2019), Harell (2017) and Stienstra (2018) have explored the critical intersections of race, gender, and disability, the detrimental impact of xenophobia and Islamophobia on disabled refugees in Canada has been alarmingly neglected.

Xenophobia thrives in nations that propagate the unfounded dominant narrative that refugees are dangerous and pose a threat to a nation's cultural identity. The construction of an exclusive national identity plays a significant role in shaping how xenophobia affects newcomers to Canada. Historically, xenophobia has been rooted in a fear of outsiders; however, it has evolved to encompass the notion that the dominant culture of the Global North is superior to that of the Global South (Yakushko, 2009). Even racialized persons born in a country or who have resided there for many years may face xenophobia simply because they are not white and perceived as foreign because of their race, ethnicity, or culture. This xenophobic sentiment was echoed in Donald Trump's 'Make America Great Again' campaign, which alluded to a desire for an all-white America and a return to white supremacist American culture.

Xenophobia is not simply a belief of mistrust and fear of the foreign other; it manifests in public policies, legislation, and institutional practices that isolate and ostracize refugees. For instance, the American Muslim ban prohibited immigrants and refugees from Muslim-majority countries from entering the United States under the pretext of national security threats (Elkassem et al., 2018). Such policies stem from the unfounded idea that Islam breeds hate and that all Muslims have the inherent potential to be terrorists, which furthers the dehumanization of refugees, exacerbating their marginalization.

Similarly, Islamophobia is a systematic process of othering that breeds 'a biased and discriminatory view of Muslims' (Smith, 2019, p. 2) and hostility towards Arabs (Beydoun, 2016). A 2015 survey by the Angus Reid Institute found that Canadians harbourd the most negative feelings and fear towards Muslims compared to other faith groups (Angus Reid, 2015). A 2016 survey of Muslims in Canada conducted by the Environics Institute concluded that 33 per cent of Canadian Muslims experienced discrimination based on their religious and ethnic identities (Neuman, 2016). These experiences occurred in various settings, including at schools and places of employment, and involved daily microaggressions in public spaces. The rise of Islamophobia has resulted both from the historical oppression of Muslims and Arabs in the Global North and from white supremacists' political and economic interests (Bukar, 2020). Since 2016, alt-right media outlets have become increasingly popular, and anti-Muslim, anti-immigrant, and anti-refugee messaging has become more visible to Canadian audiences (Wilkins-Laflamme, 2018). However, Islamophobic sentiment does not only come from white supremacists or far-right-wing groups or platforms. In a case study of media coverage of Muslims by *Maclean's* magazine, Awan et al. (2007) detail the Islamophobic content published by the magazine between 2005 and 2007. The analysis reveals how the mainstream magazine promotes Islamophobia by representing Muslims as violent threats to western democracy and human rights values.

While the term Islamophobia suggests a fear of Muslims and Islam, Bullock and Zhou (2017) argue that it goes beyond an irrational fear; instead, '[t]he contemporary phenomenon of anti-Muslim hate, unfortunately named "Islamophobia" (because it is an ideology of hate rather than a "fear" of Muslims akin to an analogous fear of, say, spiders), is a neo-Orientalist discourse of Islam/Muslims that marks ... the hegemonic view of Muslims as portrayed in Western media' (p. 4). While Islamophobia is not synonymous with Orientalism, Beck et al. (2017) contend that understanding Orientalism is essential to disrupt Islamophobia. Rahman (2017) connects the concept of Islamophobia to Said's notion of Orientalism and describes Islamophobia as a process of othering Muslims.

Within the context of Islamophobia, xenophobia, and ableism, disabled Syrian refugees in Canada face a myriad of intersecting oppressions. Kimberlé Crenshaw, a civil rights advocate who coined the term intersectionality in the 1980s, suggests that intersectionality involves analyzing how different axes of oppression intersect and compound each other (Crenshaw, 1991). Crenshaw illustrates the term's relevance with an example of the multidimensionality of black women's experiences in the United States, specifically within the context of police gun violence. She describes how black men and boys whom police officers have killed have received some media attention, and names such as Jimmy Atchison, and Willie McCoy have been published and shared in the media (Crenshaw, 2016). In contrast, Black women like Korryn Gaines and Michelle Cusseaux, who was also a victim of police violence, remain largely unknown to the public, their stories often silenced or ignored (Crenshaw, 2016).

Our lived stories are not framed around a single axis of social division. They are shaped by many factors that influence each other at different times and in different ways, creating individualized experiences (Hill Collins and Bilge, 2016). Contrary to viewing gender, race, and class as separate and distinct social categories, the concept of intersectionality assumes that intersectional identities are interconnected (Crenshaw, 1995). However, intersectionality is not about identifying sameness and difference or stacking identities and oppressions (Crenshaw, 1998, 2016; Dhamoon, 2011). Instead, distinctive identities emerge from experiences of intersectionality and result in individuals experiencing complex and unique oppressions. In this way, an intersectional framework can identify and confront social and political structures that reinforce marginalization.

For example, Berne et al. (2018) highlight 10 principles of disability justice, proposing a conceptual framework that recognizes our bodies' diversity, uniqueness, and beauty. Of these principles, the first is intersectionality. An intersectional approach considers the historical, social, and political contexts and recognizes the individual's unique experience based on the intersection of all relevant grounds. This approach allows the experience of discrimination, based on the confluence of the grounds involved, to be recognized and remedied (Ontario Human Rights Commission, 2001). For example, in its policy on ableism, the Ontario Human Rights Commission (2016, p. 19) acknowledges that '[t]he concept of intersectional discrimination recognizes that people's lives involve multiple interrelated identities and that marginalization and exclusion based on Human Code grounds may exist because of how these identities intersect'.

In this way, disabled refugees may experience marginalization based on ableism or xenophobia and the intersection of racism, ableism, and xenophobia, amongst other interrelated oppressions. Berne (2015) explains how the framework is necessary to capture the intersectional oppressions of all disabled persons, not just white, middle-class, and heterosexual disabled persons:

> While a concrete and radical move forward toward justice, the disability rights movement simultaneously invisibilized the lives of people who lived at intersecting junctures of oppression – disabled people of colour, immigrants with disabilities, trans and gender non-conforming people with disabilities, people with disabilities who are houseless, people with disabilities who are incarcerated, people with disabilities who have had their ancestral lands stolen, amongst others.

Some disability scholarship that seeks to move away from biomedical definitions has nonetheless failed to interrogate the colonial and capitalist foundations of ableism, thereby perpetuating a discourse that centers white, Western experiences and ignores intersectional perspectives. Migration scholars have also ignored how refugees may occupy multiple social locations within a host country and outside of it (Anthias, 2012). Their social locations may differ in their pre-migration, migration journey, and postmigration stages. Gangamma and Shipman (2018, p. 216) propose the term 'transnational intersectionality', which 'alerts us to the possible ways in which processes of power and marginalization overlap, evolve, complicate, and sometimes contradict across national contexts in the lives of refugees'.

Just as concepts like gendered racism (Essed, 1991), gendered Islamophobia (Zine, 2004), and racist ableism (Gorman, forthcoming) reveal powerful intersections of oppression, the narratives shared in this study underscore the inseparable nature of these intersecting forms of discrimination. When the experiences and impacts of disablement and displacement are treated separately, the stories of disabled refugees are not only disregarded; they are rewritten. By utilizing a transnational lens and critically examining concepts of intersectional oppressions, citizenship, and othering, this research contributes to a new way of understanding 'racist ableism', a form of ableism that directly and systemically intersects with racism. Gorman shares how 'racist ableism' prompts us to consider the perspectives of anti-racist and transnational feminist scholars, who highlight unique manifestations of racialized gender oppression that affect specific groups disproportionately. This concept illuminates how ableism is not only reinforced by racial biases but also perpetuates systems of white supremacy. As articulated by Gorman (ibid.), 'racist ableism is part of a white supremacist settler logic that affords the possibility of reclaimed white privilege and belonging for some disabled subjects (subjects who are more proximate to white middle-class respectability) in part through the othering and/or erasure of BIPOC [black, Indigenous, and people of colour] disabled subjects'.

The stories presented in Chapter Five underscore the necessity of acknowledging and understanding the complex intersection of xenophobia and ableism experienced by the participants. Disabled refugees face unique and compounded challenges that cannot be fully understood through the lens of either xenophobia or ableism alone. The concept of xenophobic ableism, which I propose, sheds light on how these two forms of oppression intersect and intensify each other, thereby compounding the hardships faced by disabled refugees.

Xenophobic ableism refers to the way xenophobia exacerbates ableism, leading to a heightened level of discrimination and marginalization for individuals who are both disabled and displaced. For example, a disabled refugee might face barriers in accessing healthcare not only due to their disability but also because of language barriers, cultural misunderstandings, and prejudiced attitudes towards refugees. This intersectional oppression manifests in various ways, from exclusionary policies and practices to harmful everyday social interactions, all of which contribute to the systemic barriers that disabled refugees encounter. Recognizing xenophobic ableism as a distinct and intersectional form of oppression provides deeper insight into the intricate and often overlooked narratives of disablement and displacement shared by the participants. This lens allows for a more nuanced examination of the multifaceted impact of oppression on disabled refugees. It highlights how their experiences of discrimination are not just additive but interwoven, creating a complex web of exclusion that affects their access to resources, social inclusion, and overall well-being.

CHAPTER 5
Sharing real-life stories

The real stories of the participants emerge more clearly within the backdrop of the theoretical underpinnings discussed in Chapter Four. The critical perspective provides a more nuanced understanding of the storytellers' intersecting identities, experiences, and oppressions. The meticulous data analysis led me to place specific stories and segments of storied experiences into 11 themes. These thematic sections are not intended to exist alone; they are interconnected pieces woven together to unveil both authentic individual narratives and collective concerns.

Stories of disablement

Each story shared with me was complex, multifaceted, and layered. Disability as an identity, as a social construction, a physical impairment, a medical condition, and as a direct result of war and structural violence were all ideas entwined into the conversations. Identifying as a disabled person was never tricky for Amal. Her story, which reflects her lifelong struggle for inclusion and acceptance within an ableist society, centres around disablement. Growing up disabled and as a wheelchair user, Amal was subjected to ableist assumptions that she could never succeed in school or get a decent job. She was always told that no one would want to marry her and that she could never bear children. Despite the systemic ableist environmental and attitudinal barriers surrounding her, Amal performed well in school, found a meaningful job, fell in love, married the man of her dreams, and had children. However, when her first child was born with a developmental disability, societal attitudes turned even more hostile. She recounted angrily an encounter where a visitor came to her house and insensitively remarked on the increasing number of disabled individuals in her family, implying a curse. Wiping away her tears, she repeated his words that continue to haunt her, 'There was one, then there were two, and now there are three', referring to the increasing number of disabled persons in her family.

Amal opened up about the ableist stigma attached to being a disabled parent. While her experiences are discussed within the context of Syria, the misconceptions about parenting for disabled persons are echoed globally. Parenting with a disability is often met with the notion that parents must possess the physical, financial, and emotional independence to care for their children adequately (Olsen and Clarke, 2003; Parchomiuk, 2014). Amal emphasized that it was not her disability or her child's disability that posed the most significant challenge but rather the societal scorn and judgment endured by her family. Despite all of this, it was not until the war broke out that Amal truly grasped the extent to which disabled persons are devalued. She expressed how disabled persons were the last to receive aid and the last to be evacuated to a safe area following military attacks.

She further explained how, even in Canada, disabled persons are the last to be evacuated in emergency situations. She recounted how difficult it was to get accessible housing when she arrived in Canada. Finally, after being placed in an accessible apartment, she experienced an incident that starkly reminded her of her social status. One day, the fire alarm went off in her apartment building, and it took her back to the traumatic experiences of being left behind in Syria. Amal scoffed and shared how she was the last to vacate the building since she required assistance to come down the stairs, which means she was likely to be the first to die in a fire. 'Imagine, I escaped war to be left in a burning building.' Amal drew parallels between living with a disability in Syria and Canada. In both countries, her life has less value. She is undeserving of protection, dignity, and the most basic care.

Like Amal, Hassan also shared his journey of raising disabled children in Syria. Since their early years, Hassan's children encountered difficulties with traditional learning and socializing in school. Hassan worked closely with teachers and therapists to provide his kids with the necessary support so they could learn and make friends. However, the economic sanctions and political circumstances meant that his family did not receive adequate medical attention or support, including the medication his wife required during pregnancy. It was not until Hassan resettled in Canada that he gained insight into the genetic nature of his children's medical conditions. Before they arrived in Canada, Hassan encountered various medical professionals who were unable to diagnose his children's conditions accurately. He received conflicting advice regarding the nature of their conditions and the appropriate strategies and supports that could help them:

> I went to a lot of doctors; nobody knew what was wrong with them in Syria. Okay the second child came and then third child came along. We went to another doctor to deliver, a good doctor to deliver the third child and they said that it has nothing to do with the way he was born. Then we got pregnant with the fourth child as the doctor said it's not that she [wife] will have the same problem and the fourth child did have the same condition.

Upon learning about his children's diagnoses, Hassan began researching treatments. He explained that his children were born with a genetic condition that required prenatal medical treatment and early intervention. In Canada, newborns undergo routine screening for approximately 25 genetic conditions shortly after birth (Newborn Screening Ontario, 2021). Hassan's children's condition falls within the spectrum of those that are identifiable and likely treatable if detected early. Hassan expressed how the lack of access to proper medical care in both Syria and the host country his family sought asylum in had a detrimental impact on his children's development and well-being.

Marwa had a similar experience as Hassan, having been given inconsistent information from doctors in Syria and Canada. Two of her kids were experiencing delays in walking and talking from a young age and often complained of muscle weakness and pain. Marwa received reassurance from doctors in Syria that her children had a curable disease. When she arrived in Canada, Marwa thought doctors would rush to provide the necessary medication to cure her children's condition. However, she was taken aback to discover that obtaining medical tests or specialist appointments in Canada could take several months or even years. She had difficulty finding a primary care physician and was frequently turned away from hospital emergency rooms because her children's conditions were chronic, not acute. It was not until over a year after she arrived in Canada that Marwa received the disheartening news that there was no medication or cure available for her children's progressive conditions. They would eventually lose the ability to walk and require assistance with their activities of daily living such as feeding and toileting. This revelation left her feeling disillusioned and uncertain about the future well-being of her children:

> I started to see doctors around. I met the neurology doctor after six months after my arrival and they referred me to the children's hospital for my two daughters. Well, they started to do some tests and they did genetic tests, and it took another six months for it to come. I got the results and they said it's not what we thought, it's something close to it. It's malformation in the genes. Unfortunately, they told us this disease doesn't have a treatment and that there might be some tests or treatment in the future.

Unlike Marwa, Hassan, and Amal, whose children were born with disabilities, Omar shared a different experience of disablement. His child's disability was acquired as a direct result of armed conflict. Omar recounted how his son's condition stemmed from the severe shortage of essential medical supplies, notably oxygen, resulting from the sanctions imposed on Syria. Furthermore, strict military curfews severely limited access to humanitarian aid and the movement of civilians, including healthcare workers. The ambulance simply could not reach Omar's area in time to help his son. He painfully recalled feeling helpless while witnessing his child struggle for breath:

> My son, he had lack of oxygen when he was born and then due to the war, they couldn't get his medication and the care he needs. So now he developed a damage to his brain.

Like Omar, Muna also recounted the direct horrors of the conflict that were inflicted on her child. She described fleeing an area in Syria ravaged by poisonous chemicals and remains deeply troubled about the harmful aftermath of those toxins on her family. Since escaping Syria, she has advocated for the treatment of her child's condition:

> When he was three, we took him to a doctor in Lebanon, and the doctor said the child has a high metal and high toxicity. It could be a result of chemical poison they said.

Muna shared how the doctors in Lebanon were aware of the atrocities of war that led to chemical poisoning. However, when she arrived in Canada, she found that doctors were sceptical of her story. Not only did they dismiss her family's transnational stories of disability, but they also relied strictly on the (Global North) standardized medical assessments and protocols for developmental disabilities. Despite her ongoing efforts to convey the realities of her son's condition, Canadian healthcare workers expressed their inability to verify the information she shared and only addressed her child's immediate health concerns, effectively rewriting her narrative.

What is the impact of chemical weapons on paediatric disabilities? In a 2021 submission, the Syria Justice and Accountability Centre identified the need for further research on the immediate and long-term impacts of chemical weapons on children and pleaded for international medical organizations to make this research a priority. Hakeem and Jabri (2015) underscore the importance of investigating the long-term health effects of chemical weapons in Syria, particularly on pregnant women and their children, who may experience lifelong health conditions due to exposure to toxic substances.

Muna's story, like the other participants, requires an acknowledgement and validation of her experiences of disablement that extend beyond the confines of a doctor's office or a medical textbook. It requires one to think past a dominant narrative that separates displacement from disablement. It reflects a lived experience of disability that cannot be fully captured through medical diagnoses alone. For example, the chemical attacks in Syria not only led to civilian strife, disability, and death, but were compounded by international responses from the Global North, which, through arms sales and missile attacks, further disabled, maimed, and killed the civilian population.

Stories of a disabling Syria

The stories of disablement were intertwined with the stories of a disabling Syrian society. Participants reminisced about Syria before the war when they were not displaced or refugees. Their narratives highlighted Syria's rich history, breathtaking landscapes, tight-knit interdependent communities, and dynamic culture with great food, music, art, and much more. They discussed their experiences at school and work, spending time with family and friends, and their aspirations for a prosperous future. They all shared how much they love their country. They spoke about their cultural and faith communities and described their hopes and dreams for the future. They all discussed the war as a point in time that changed everything, and they all spoke about leaving Syria to protect their families. Muhammad said:

> After the war broke out, things spiralled out of control. Jobs were gone, homes destroyed, infrastructure broken, and lives lost.

Much like Muhammad, other participants recounted their escape from Syria out of necessity, driven by the need to protect their families, particularly their children, from the ravages of war. They describe how the armed conflict thrust them into the unfamiliar role of refugees, a status they never anticipated or chose willingly. Rather, it was the dire circumstances of the war that forced them into this new identity. Jahan, a private sponsor I conversed with, offered insights into the prevailing narrative surrounding refugees, emphasizing that portraying them as 'lucky' to be in Canada overlooks the harsh realities they face. She stressed that seeking refuge is not a matter of choice but of sheer survival: coming to Canada is their last resort for safety and security.

This choice to leave Syria to survive was shared through powerful statements by several participants:

> "I left Syria because of the way it was difficult with the war, there was no work and no security. I was afraid for my family. We did not feel safe, everything was so difficult."
>
> —Sarah

> "I was afraid that I was going to lose one of my kids in the war. I could not lose any more and I could not lose my children."
>
> —Muna

> "My kids wanted to go out of Syria because of the traumatizing things they saw under explosions. They wanted to live. I wanted them to live."
>
> —Halima

Beyond the immediate fear of death, the conflict in Syria also led to widespread unemployment, starvation, extreme poverty, the demolition of homes, businesses, and places of worship, physical injuries, psychological trauma, and a severe lack of access to healthcare and social support systems. In essence, the war altered every facet of their existence. Muhammad and Amal shed light on the profound economic challenges they faced within Syria, in neighbouring host countries, and eventually in Canada. They recount experiences of financial insecurity and psychological stress that plagued them at every stage of their displacement journey. Amal described the devastating impact of losing her and her husband's jobs, leaving them unable to provide for their basic needs. This financial strain hindered their capacity to care for themselves and their children:

> The war destroyed my family home and my husband's business and with my son having a disability there was no support for him. One day, my child got really sick. We did not even have money to take him even to the hospital. Our neighbour came and he took the child from us. He ran to the hospital with him, and he paid for everything. And that was... ugh that hurt. And we were very embarrassed that we weren't able to provide our son with whatever he needed. That's when we decided to get out of Syria, and we would try to find a place where they could provide for his needs.

Omar was one participant who did not describe the devastation or destruction in Syria in detail. Instead, he looked at me and said, 'I need not tell you a lot about the difficulties in the war because mostly we all know about it. For us, it was real'. Despite my scepticism about the extent to which we are truly aware of the authentic narratives of the Syrian war, due to biased media coverage and political censorship shaping a dominant narrative, I refrained from pressing Omar to expand. His statement led me to ponder Clandinin's (2013) notions of retelling and reliving stories. I thought about how pain is often revisited through the pervasive imagery and rhetoric that comes with sharing stories. Moreover, I considered the tendency to overlook the trauma inherent in recounting one's own experiences, as highlighted by Saleh (2019). Sharing narratives that diverge from the dominant discourse entails more than simply presenting an alternative viewpoint. It necessitates the arduous task of defending and substantiating one's story, particularly stories of hardship and suffering. Omar's assertion that the story was real served as a powerful reminder that the stories shared by the participants were not fabricated; they were authentic reflections of lived experiences.

Stories of difficult journeys

The pain and suffering echoed in the participants' stories were not just about their child's disability and the impact of the war on their family. Their stories involved the distressing physical journeys of displacement, the squalid conditions and dangerous lengthy stays in refugee camps, the dehumanizing ordeal of seeking asylum with immense policing (specifically around disability), and the horrors that came with the forced reallocation of many generations. Stories of refugees are often portrayed simply as leaving one place and arriving at another (Issari et al., 2021). Discussions of displacement and asylum seeking frequently fail to capture the full extent of forced migration, which includes the means and conditions of transportation and the profound impact of a dangerous journey.

In 2015, my sister Fatema was volunteering at a Syrian refugee camp in Leros, Greece. During her time there, she would send my family emails about her experiences and the devastating accounts she witnessed. Fatema described hundreds of refugees arriving on small overcrowded boats along the coast. Some endured the exhausting, perilous journey. Some were barely alive upon arrival. Fatema described how the journey out of Syria resembles a gruelling survival-of-the-fittest test that many refugees, especially children, could not withstand. I pulled up one of her emails from her time in Leros, dated January 1st, 2016, in which she wrote to my family:

> They were on the boat, cold and wet for days without food. We gave them three biscuits and water when they arrived. Only three biscuits! The two girls were soaking wet because no one would get them a pad, so I asked one of the officers if I could take them to the bathroom, helped get her a change of clothes. She spoke a bit of English, so I was able to understand that her brother was also not well – looked at his fingers that had gone all blue and purple – so the medics were allowed to take him to the makeshift tent to get some assistance.

The conditions Fatema described in her emails highlight the authentic narratives of displacement and disablement. As I sifted through them, I encountered accounts of the mistreatment endured by refugees along their paths of forced displacement. These included stories of strict monitoring of daily activities, numerous violent security checkpoints, hours spent waiting in queues for food, endless paperwork for refugee applications, limited access to essential resources such as medical aid, and a discriminatory selection procedure that determined who could advance in the asylum-seeking process based on physical abilities, age, gender, and education level. Those who were deemed able could proceed, while others faced further obstacles. While this selection process for who gets asylum may seem arbitrary within dominant discourse, I recognized that the narratives within Fatema's emails exemplified instances of intersecting oppressions, othering, and transnational disablement. Although I had not critically analysed these concepts when initially reading her emails years earlier, delving deeper into disablement within the context of displacement prompted me to question why such powerful intersectional issues were ignored within the asylum-seeking process.

All the families I spoke with sought refuge in neighbouring countries before coming to Canada, including Egypt, Lebanon, Türkiye, and Jordan. They all believed that seeking refuge in neighbouring countries would be far safer and more promising than the situation in Syria. Many participants reported that these host countries' economic, political, and social situations were highly challenging for refugees, especially since they could only come with the bags they could carry. Muhammad, for example, expressed how the conditions in Jordan were just as bad as those in Syria. He felt helpless. He struggled to provide for his family because he could not secure employment. Muhammad described the situation as feeling 'completely powerless', reliant on the resources in the refugee camp where he was placed. Furthermore, the camp was not wheelchair accessible, which meant that Muhammad's child was confined to a small bed, which led to a significant regression in his child's mobility and social skills.

Other participants shared their experiences of extreme poverty in their host country, including food and housing insecurity. There was also a looming threat of persecution and imprisonment as they were not yet accepted as refugees, which made them particularly vulnerable, lacking the social, economic, and political protections afforded to citizens. They also did not have the family and community support in the host country that they did in Syria. Muna recounted the financial difficulties her family faced:

> It was one of the most difficult part[s] of my life. Uh, we didn't have any money to fulfil any of our needs.

Marwa believed she would be greeted with significant support upon arrival in the host country, given the common understanding that forcibly displaced persons could not travel with their belongings. 'We only had the clothes on our backs', she recounted, illustrating the stark connection between poverty and displacement. Marwa explained how her family's financial situation meant she could not afford to send her kids to the private school for disabled children. Consequently, they were deprived of educational opportunities, compounding their learning difficulties:

> When the war started, we went to Lebanon. I was hoping that the medical care is better in Lebanon than Syria. I tried to send them [kids with disabilities] to school but they didn't accept them. The private schools were very expensive, so I kept them home and they didn't go to school there. I started my journey, and I had depression, and it was really hard for me.

While participants faced many obstacles in the journey to the host country, the trip to Canada proved to be even more difficult. This journey involved navigating complex immigration processes, overcoming bureaucratic hurdles, and enduring lengthy wait times to be processed for resettlement. Moreover, the emotional toll of leaving behind familiar surroundings, culture, language, and loved ones and the uncertainty of starting anew in an unfamiliar land made the flight to Canada even more daunting.

Mainstream media narratives that Canadians were exposed to made it sound like Syrian refugees all rejoiced when they landed at the airport, being welcomed by dignitaries and sponsors, overcome with feelings of relief and gratitude. For example, a 2015 *Globe and Mail* article reads: 'Relieved and exhausted, refugees arrived late in the evening to be met by the Prime Minister, Ontario's Premier and refugee sponsors' (*Globe and Mail*, 2015). Contrary to this perception of widespread support and celebration, Sarah shared how difficult her migration to Canada was:

> Coming to Canada was a horrible, horrible experience. I tried to get Hussain [child with a disability] in the airplane and he was crying and screaming and hitting us all and hitting people even around him ... it was a disaster. And the people around us were really irritated that we couldn't do anything about it.

Halima also shared her experience of feeling anxious and overwhelmed on the airplane and struggling to connect with fellow passengers and airport staff. Upon boarding, she keenly sensed the judgment from others and their apparent lack of empathy, particularly towards disabled children. Halima's children required additional support; she shared how they were tired and scared. As a mother, I could not help but recall my own experiences of travelling alone with my two young children, facing disapproving glances from fellow passengers when they cried, and feeling hesitant to ask for assistance, especially as a visibly Muslim woman. What Halima shared, however, was far more than unpleasant experiences; it left her traumatized:

> The journey was difficult. The trip it was super difficult. It was like we suffered more than other people. The kids weren't able also to carry their bags or do anything. So, it was so super, super difficult for us. And it was a long, long trip. Every one of them [children] needs to go to the washroom. They need me to go with them and it was really difficult. No one was helping us, even when we asked for help.

As I listened to Halima's narrative, I could hear notes of anger in her voice as she described how she could not leave her other scared children with strangers when taking one child to the toilet, especially when they looked at her like she was a monster. Halima anticipated the airplane ride to be an exhilarating adventure reminiscent of what she had seen portrayed on television. Instead, she was met with stares and scorn from fellow passengers, making her family feel unsafe, unwelcome, and out of place. Sarah shared a similar experience: she had nothing to distract her son on the airplane or tools to help him remain calm during take-off. He shouted throughout the journey, and the flight attendants increasingly became upset with her for not keeping him quiet. Sarah's story highlights the need for flight attendants to be aware of diverse experiences and learn to treat and support disabled persons and their families with dignity and respect.

Marwa also shared her fears about travelling in an airplane for the first time. She discloses how, at no point in time, when filling out her paperwork or when preparing for the migration journey, was the process of travelling to Canada explained to her family. She did not know what to expect. For example, she did not know how long the journey would be, who would be there to greet her family when they arrived, or what kind of support they would receive once they landed:

> I was so scared, I was terrified, I was coming to the unknown. My first time travelling in an airplane, I was so scared.

As they described their migration journeys, the participants echoed the experience of having a disabled child who required additional support and having their rights as disabled children realized. They shared how their children needed to be carried or pushed in a stroller or wheelchair and how they required specific help with essential tasks like feeding and toileting. Participants shared their numerous difficulties supporting their children during the long car rides, dangerous boat trips, and exhausting flights to Canada. These journeys were emotionally and physically taxing, and throughout the process, they were consumed with concern about their own safety and the safety of their families.

Stories of trauma

Stories of trauma permeated every dialogue I had with the storytellers. They narrated harrowing experiences of trauma during the conflict, throughout their displacement journeys, and upon their arrival in Canada. Participants spoke of the constant exposure to bombings, the immense grief they experienced having lost friends and family, and the mass destruction of infrastructure, all of which left deep emotional scars. Upon reaching Canada, their sense of safety was often overshadowed by the lingering effects of their traumatic experiences, as well as the challenges of adapting to a new and unfamiliar environment. They shared how these traumatic experiences have profound short and long-term impacts on themselves and their families, affecting their mental health, physical well-being, and overall quality of life. 'Do they know what we went through? I wonder if they know about what we went through', Omar asked rhetorically, his voice shaking. He paused for a moment, then said:

> We had no electricity, no water, no food, nothing there, and no hospitals, and for me, so I couldn't look after my leg. I couldn't walk properly and get help for my family.

As I quietly listened to Omar, I could not help but feel that many people may not fully understand what he and the other participants endured. Since we are often exposed to a dominant narrative, Omar's story may be unfamiliar, as authentic narratives of disablement and displacement are frequently overlooked or overshadowed by more palatable versions. Despite extensive coverage of the Syrian war in the news and documented accounts detailing its impact on communities, the dominant narrative prevails. As discussed in Chapter Two, this dominant narrative fails to acknowledge the complexity of human experiences and the enduring effects of trauma on refugees.

Reflecting on my profession as an occupational therapist in Canada, I have come to realize significant gaps in my education and training, partly due to the limited exposure to non-dominant stories of disablement and displacement. In the case studies I examined during my training, the Canadian experience was primarily presented in a uniform way. While my undergraduate studies covered subjects like health policy, equity studies, and bioethics, there was little emphasis on understanding the profound impacts of individual and collective trauma and the material and economic conditions affecting disabled refugees in Canada. Even during my master's in occupational therapy, where the focus shifted towards occupational performance, occupational justice, and client and family-centred care, there was a lack of attention given to the systemic impacts of social determinants of health and disability within displaced populations. Intersectional experiences and oppressions, as well as the effects of intergenerational trauma, were all overlooked in the coursework, case studies, and clinical placements.

Looking back over the years, the absence of critical discussions and reflections throughout my schooling is alarming. Despite attending public elementary, middle, and high schools in Kitchener, Ontario, I was never taught about Canada's institutionalized oppression, like the history of slavery in Canada, the forced assimilation of immigrants and refugees, and the cruel inhumane treatment of disabled persons in psychiatric hospitals. Moreover, I received no instruction on Canada's settler-colonial history, including the mass killing and mistreatment of Indigenous peoples, the forced separation of children from their families through residential schools (including one that was less than an hour away from my elementary school), and the erasure of the culture of brown and black populations. Throughout my schooling, there was a profound lack of non-dominant local and transnational histories and narratives to comprehend real-life experiences, oppressions, and systemic settler-colonial societal issues, let alone identify potential solutions. 'Our profession is supposed to be culturally responsive and trauma-informed! (Government of Canada, 2018)' Salma, one of the settlement workers, exclaimed, continuing:

> But nobody is talking about trauma, and in fact, in most of the cases we hear, not only are they not talking about trauma, or intergenerational trauma, but when people bring up trauma, whether in schools or at doctors' appointments, they are told they are in a different place now!

We cannot effectively discuss trauma if we ignore the historical and ongoing systems that produce and perpetuate it. Halima explained how the pain and trauma she experienced in Syria gets relived in Canada in different ways. She described how the memories of her experiences, once thought left behind, are often triggered by various interactions in Canada in both subtle and overt ways. Halima explained how sensory experiences like the sounds at the dentist's office or the school bell negatively impact her children. She has no way of explaining how trauma is manifested in all aspects of her daily life to all the many service providers and professionals she meets:

> It is traumatizing. I feel like I am often back in the same pain, the same trauma and because we stayed there in this terrible situation for two years. So, I sometimes feel like I am back in the same pain that I had before. But my oldest one is giving me a really hard time. He's not accepting anything, even his dentist appointment. I took the appointment and then when the appointment came, he doesn't want to go, and he doesn't want to do it. He is scared. I cannot force him, so I cannot do anything for him. He is afraid.

As a settlement worker who interacts with refugees daily and advocates for their needs, Yasmine shed light on the inconsistent perception and treatment of trauma by healthcare and educational professionals. She emphasized that the experiences refugees endure profoundly affect their physical and mental health, often in ways that require specialized care. 'The refugee experience is significantly misunderstood', she emphasized. Refugees are frequently lumped together with immigrants despite the crucial distinction between the two. Unlike immigrants, refugees are individuals seeking protection from imminent harm, violence, and devastation in their home countries (CCD, 2012).

This critical misunderstanding and lack of recognition of the refugee experience have significant ramifications for Sarah. She articulated how she grapples with reliving the trauma of her past daily. This ongoing ordeal has manifested into a chronic medical condition. She experiences debilitating anxiety and high blood pressure, which significantly impacts her life in Canada. Despite her physical distance from the source of her trauma, its effects continue to echo through her daily existence, highlighting the urgent need for a more empathetic and trauma-informed approach to healthcare and support services for refugees:

> I'm hoping that nothing would happen to me. My heart condition is not good. I need to be able to take care of my kids and do everything. Because this happened all because of the stress and the fear, feeling, and everything that I have been through.

For Sarah, the narratives she shared during our conversation only scratch the surface of her harrowing journey. As she wiped away her tears, she smiled and said:

> One day I may be able to do something like write something and express what I did in my life, someone might want to read it. People don't know what we have been through.

I cannot help but ask, what if Sarah does share her journey, but it is dismissed? What if she speaks up and her voice is silenced? Families I work with at SMILE Canada often tell me that they have shared their stories of trauma multiple times with multiple professionals, only to have their experiences overlooked. Richard Mollica coined the term 'the trauma story' after establishing the first refugee clinic in the United States. Mollica documented narratives of trauma from Cambodian women, and his research led to the recognition of four key elements found within the stories. Firstly, the details are critical and cannot be overlooked; they form the backbone of the narrative. Secondly, cultural context shapes how individuals experience and communicate their trauma. Thirdly, each story reveals layers of insight and understanding as it unfolds. Finally, the relationship between the storyteller and the listener is pivotal in how these stories are shared and understood (Mollica, 2001).

Stories of Canadian struggles

After settling in Canada, the narratives of disablement persisted for the participants, marked by ongoing exclusion, isolation, and intersecting forms of oppression. Sarah's experiences at the hotel shelter exemplify this reality. While others were able to enjoy their time once they arrived at a safe shelter, Sarah's family could not even leave their hotel room due to her child's social and behavioural needs. What was meant to be a period of relief and hope instead felt isolating and unsupported. Sarah found herself overwhelmed with anxiety and doubt, questioning the decision to move her family to Canada. Sarah's frustration was compounded by the hotel staff's insensitivity towards her child's disability and her family's situation. She felt the staff fell short of providing the necessary support despite her family's apparent need for understanding and assistance:

> Okay, well everybody in the hotel were having fun. They were going to the swimming pool and eating in the restaurant. But we had to go through a lot of trouble because we couldn't go to the restaurant because my son was giving them a hard time. He used to hit them there so we were only allowed to eat in the room and even the elevator, we wouldn't get in there. The staff did not help us.

As Sarah shared her story, I wondered if the staff at the settlement agency and hotel shelter understood the critical needs of disabled children and their families, and their legal right to accommodations. I wondered if they had been educated or trained in supporting disabled children and children with physical and psychological trauma. Marwa's experience further fuelled this reflection. She expressed a deep longing to return to Syria shortly after arriving in Canada, despite the encouragement from her private sponsors to embrace the benefits of her new and 'safe' environment. Marwa's story reveals a profound longing for her homeland's community culture, where neighbours were akin to family. Despite being urged to appreciate the opportunities in Canada, she struggles to feel a sense of belonging and misses the warmth and familiarity of her Syrian community:

> After a month, I was so depressed, I was talking to my husband, I wanted to go back. The sponsor told me the advantages of being in Canada. But I was depressed. I didn't speak the language and secondly the Arabic culture – we always have neighbours, and we are so close together and I came here, and I was disconnected from everybody. There is no culture like that here, neighbours aren't talking to each other.

Sarah's feelings about wanting to return to Syria highlight the difficulties she faced upon arrival in Canada and the need to listen to her share her experience. Her story underscores the necessity for organizations and those involved in the resettlement process to be attuned to the diverse experiences and barriers displaced families face, ensuring they feel genuinely welcomed and supported in their new environment. Despite the promise of safety and opportunity in Canada, Hajra also shared how she faces ongoing obstacles:

> Here [in Canada], we saw other struggles than we saw in Syria. We are having other struggles. All my years here [in Canada] are full of struggles.

Dalia, the eldest participant in the study, recounted the difficulties she faced upon arrival in Canada, as her husband brought her lunch on a tray. 'He's an amazing cook', she boasted. Her smile quickly faded as she began to describe their asylum-seeking story. Upon arrival, they received essential resources such as food, shelter, and clothing from a local settlement agency. However, what became painfully evident was the oversight regarding Dalia's disability. Her disability-related needs were disregarded. She did not receive the crucial rehabilitation services, therapies, or adaptive equipment she required. The settlement agency also did not provide any information on disability-related resources or direct Dalia to any centre for accessible transportation or home modifications. As time passed and the refugee agency's support dwindled, Dalia and her husband were left to fend for themselves. She shared her yearning for the emotional, social, and financial support her adult children could provide. She described how her children's Canadian visa applications were all rejected, leaving Dalia and her husband abandoned and lonely. In addition to grappling with the emotional toll of being separated from her children and prevented from meeting her grandchildren in person, Dalia also expressed concerns about her husband's health: 'His health is not good, but we care for each other'. The thought of something happening to him weighs heavily on her mind:

> I need my son to help me. What if something happened to my husband? I am going to be left alone. I cannot do anything by myself.

Dalia discussed the many social and environmental differences between Syria and Canada, highlighting one notable challenge: the harsh Canadian winters, a climate very different from the milder weather she was accustomed to in Syria. Several other participants echoed this sentiment and described finding themselves ill-prepared for the heavy snow and extreme cold temperatures. Research by Aldiabat et al. (2021) supports these personal accounts, showing that extreme cold temperatures impact the everyday health of Syrian refugees. Halima, for example, shared how ensuring her disabled children stayed safe and warm amidst the freezing weather required considerable effort. The extra layers of clothing and winter accessories they needed added other challenges to an already tricky adjustment process:

> And well, being here in November it was winter, and here gets anyway like it's so hard for them to adjust to new temperature so they were refusing the change and specifically in winter they had to wear gloves and hats and they are not used to it. So, it was an extra. The winter was difficult. Until now my son, he does not wear gloves or a hat in the winter. Yeah, we found it really difficult to adjust and it took them a long time to adjust it specifically that they cannot leave their children alone in the house. They cannot go anywhere.

Marwa echoed this shared struggle of navigating bitter Canadian winters, especially while taking public transportation. The bitter weather compounded the challenges of finding their way and Marwa described how she and her husband often got lost and felt unsupported by those around them:

> It was really cold; I didn't have a car and it was minus 15 when I got here. We used to take a stroller with my husband

and carry big bags on my shoulders and in the cold. Every time we did this I was crying; I couldn't take it anymore. A lot of time we got lost, we didn't know where the station was. People didn't understand us and would not help us.

Even during the warmer months, using public transportation with disabled children was difficult. Naima, one of the private sponsors, explained that, like the newcomers, volunteers involved in community sponsorship need to learn about the public transportation system because they typically rely on personal vehicles. As a result, teaching newcomers how to use public transportation becomes a significant challenge. Navigating accessible public transportation is particularly tough. It involves knowing how to book and plan for wheelchair-accessible services, which do not always cross city lines, adding another layer of complexity. Public transportation systems in Canada are not adequately equipped to accommodate individuals with disabilities, leading to further obstacles for those who require these services (Comeau, 2024). Naima sighed and said:

We did not know how to do it. We were figuring it out as we were helping them [Syrian refugees] and they could probably tell.

Dalia, Sarah, and Marwa's narratives vividly paint a picture of the many challenges they faced in adapting to life in Canada. Their examples of harsh winters and the complexities of using public transportation are just a few of the hurdles disabled refugees face, which are rarely discussed within dominant narratives surrounding asylum seeking in Canada.

Stories of economic and social conditions

Every storyteller discussed financial difficulties in Canada, including the rising cost of food, gas, essential therapies, and transportation. Wilkinson and Garcea (2017) found that while many refugees obtain meaningful employment, it is not until years after they arrive. Marwa's story highlights the challenges of finding meaningful employment in Canada. Despite being legally entitled to work, Marwa struggled to secure a job that matched her skills and qualifications and paid a fair wage. Like many newcomers, Marwa and her husband invested time and money in their education and skill development in Syria. However, upon settling in Canada, they encountered language and cultural barriers that prevented them from effectively leveraging their prior experiences. As a result, they were pushed to work in a bakery, a significant departure from their previous careers. Marwa shared:

> My husband, he is a mechanic. He is a good mechanic and well known in our city. And this agency finds jobs for people, so they signed for him to work in a bakery. He could not find any job opportunity in his field, so he had to work in a bakery where he makes bread. And he is so frustrated about that he thinks he should be doing something different and take more money other than just making bread.

Marwa recalls how the same settlement agency that helped her secure a job at the bakery had previously arranged for her to work as a seamstress, sewing company emblems onto winter jackets. During her time there, Marwa felt exploited by the company due to the poor working conditions and minimal pay. Supporting five children, two of whom had significant disability-related expenses, Marwa found it challenging to make ends meet despite her hard work. She expressed frustration that her employment as a seamstress did not even allow her to purchase a single item of clothing from the company's line. This contradiction was particularly striking given that the company was often praised for supporting refugees by offering them employment opportunities. Marwa's story underscores the difference between public perception and the reality of the refugee experience, highlighting the need for better labour conditions and fair wages for refugees. This poignant acknowledgement stayed with me long after my conversation with Marwa, prompting reflection on the inequities within the workforce and the challenges faced by others like her, who contribute to producing goods for Canadians but struggle to afford them due to inappropriate compensation. It highlights the need for greater awareness and action to address systemic issues of exploitation and unfair labour practices, particularly within industries that claim to support underserved newcomer communities.

The participants also stressed the substantial financial burden associated with caring for a child with a disability, which far exceeds the costs of caring for a child without a disability, as documented by Burton and Phipps (2009). The economic implications of having a child with a disability are highlighted not only through the direct out-of-pocket expenses associated with adaptive equipment, assistive technology, therapies, respite services and medications, but also the indirect cost of lost employment and reduced financial gains. Many families caring for a child with a disability face difficult choices when balancing caregiving responsibilities with employment. Some family members may turn down job opportunities, adjust their work schedules, or even leave their jobs altogether in order to provide the care their child needs (Government of Canada. 2022). These decisions can have lasting financial and emotional impacts on the entire household. As a result, parents of children with disabilities are more likely to experience loss of wages unless they have access to employment with paid leave or flexible policies surrounding work hours (Earle and Heymann, 2012).

Many participants shared their experiences of incurring out-of-pocket expenses for essential therapies like physiotherapy, respite services, equipment such as commodes, and assistive technology. For example, using an app on an iPad to facilitate communication with their child at home is only possible if one has an iPad. Participants shared how often their child's school utilized specific tools and devices, but those remained at school. They emphasized the importance of obtaining and sustaining meaningful employment to meet these financial demands. Hassan, for instance, recounted his successful career in Syria. However, since he resettled in Canada, he has been unable to maintain employment due to his responsibilities at home caring for his wife and children. Hassan's story highlights the difficult choices faced by those who are systematically forced to prioritize caregiving duties over their professional aspirations to support their family members with disabilities:

> I was working in car mechanics and had my own shop in Syria. Like a place where I did not only work, I owned it. Well, I was working to get my family their needs but here in Canada I cannot have a job because I cannot leave my kids or my wife as she is not well, and especially in COVID also there are no schools open so there's no support at all so I cannot go and get like work and find a job. Who will take care of my children? Support is good but we need more.

> I said earlier in our conversation that I might seem selfish, but I am not being selfish, I need more help and my children need more help.

Muhammad echoes Hassan's experience of being unable to secure full-time employment due to his caregiving responsibilities at home, which require round-the-clock support. He articulated how the high cost of childcare, especially for children with disabilities and complex medical needs, presents a significant financial barrier for him. 'It simply would not work', he said. While Muhammad did not explicitly mention systemic ableism, his comments led me to reflect on the unfair reality that services for disabled children are often more expensive than services for children without disabilities. Moreover, Muhammad emphasized that it is not just unaffordable childcare expenses: essential dental and vision care services are also not publicly funded.

Furthermore, additional expenses, like a wheelchair-accessible van, are entirely out of his budget. He applied to March of Dimes Canada but is still awaiting a response. March of Dimes Canada is one organization that supports expenses for disabled persons related to home and vehicle modifications. The website reads: 'There is no guarantee for funding upon application to [the Home and Vehicle Modification Program] for accommodations related to home and vehicle modifications. Funding will depend on the dollars available and eligibility of the request' (March of Dimes Canada, 2024). Since he cannot maintain full employment, Muhammad lacks company benefits to cover these costs, further exacerbating his financial strain. Muhammad's experiences underscore the urgent need for comprehensive support systems to address the financial challenges faced by newcomer families caring for children with disabilities.

Omar shared the challenges he faces in meeting the needs of his disabled child who experiences incontinence, specifically in acquiring the specialized diapers required. These diapers are not easily found at local pharmacies and are more expensive than typical diapers. Omar explained that he needs a dedicated budget for these essential items, leading him to divert funds from other vital monthly expenses such as fuel or groceries. His situation highlights the significant financial pressure experienced by families like his, who must juggle competing priorities to ensure the well-being of their children and families.

As I listened to Omar express his concerns, I wondered if he knew non-profit organizations like SMILE Canada can assist with essential costs like diapers. However, a glaring question arises: how would participants like Omar discover additional services or funding options? How would they know whom to contact or what alternatives are available? The responsibility of who should connect families to material resources remains to be determined. Is it the duty of a family physician or a social worker? Most participants do not have access to either of these. Could it be the responsibility of teachers or settlement agencies? These questions persist without clear answers. Even when social workers and service navigators assist families, they often do not consider language, technological, or cultural needs. The applications available for specific items or services are hard to come by and difficult to complete. Sarah's experience further highlights this issue, as she mentioned needing to be directed to available support:

> Well then, nobody told me where to go or what steps to take. They [disability agency] told me that I am entitled for some things, but I don't know how to fill the applications, and they did not provide anyone to help me complete them. The country [Canada] provides some funding, services, but the thing is no one tells us that we are entitled for anything – it's mostly the individuals that are at fault.

Halima also stressed that although funding may be accessible for her child, she faces challenges understanding how to access it for necessary services and programmes. She expressed frustration, highlighting her lack of knowledge regarding where to obtain the required forms or the specific eligibility criteria for her child to qualify for disability-related funding. Halima's words conveyed her confusion and feelings of helplessness as she navigates the intricacies of the system:

> That's my problem. Yeah, nobody tells us all those about funding, about programmes or services. We don't know how to find out. Yes, like that's my problem here in Canada.

Similarly, Omar described applying for government-assisted housing five years prior, having yet to hear a single response. When he called the agency, he was told it may take another few years. 'I tried to contact social housing', he said. 'They say the wait list is very long for houses equipped for kids with special needs. Shouldn't special kids be given special consideration?' he asked sarcastically.

Stories of a pandemic survival

The interviews were conducted between 6 January and 31 July 2021, a time marked by significant challenges due to the COVID-19 pandemic. Participants faced various difficulties, including school closures, multiple lockdowns, vaccine shortages, vaccine mandates, and the virus's broader social and economic impacts (Government of Canada, 2021a). The participants felt the effects of COVID-19 both locally and globally. Some shared heartbreaking stories of losing family members to the pandemic overseas. Participants also shared concerns about access to personal protective equipment and vaccinations, especially for families in vulnerable situations, such as in crowded refugee camps. These families faced challenges in adhering to recommended protocols like physical distancing due to the crowded and unsanitary conditions. As a result, there were heightened fears about the increased risk of COVID-19 transmission and the potential for devastating consequences among already marginalized populations.

In Chapter Three, I briefly discussed my conversation with Hassan on 6 January 2021, who confronted the threat of eviction from his residence due to noise complaints about his disabled children. Hassan explained how these grievances escalated during the COVID-19 pandemic, coinciding with his children's prolonged presence at home following school closures. Like many children experiencing extended periods at home, they became increasingly restless and frustrated, leading to increased vocalizations, banging, and stomping in the apartment. The situation was exacerbated as many neighbours transitioned to remote work, remaining at home throughout the day, thus heightening sensitivity to noise disturbances.

Hassan made considerable efforts to address the situation, including keeping the windows closed to minimize noise transmission, even when ventilation was needed on hot days. He also resorted to driving his children around the neighbourhood for hours to keep them away from home. Additionally, Hassan attempted to soundproof the house by blocking doors and windows with foam sheets and placing extra rugs to dampen noise levels. Hassan paid for these modifications out of pocket:

> My kids make a lot of noise. They cannot communicate so they make these sounds. During the summer all I did was open the window and my neighbour were sitting outside, and they right away gave me a notice because the kids are being noisy. During the lockdown I am taking my kids for drives for three hours and now the mileage of the car is a lot, like 55,000 miles, and that's all I can do during the lockdown. That's because of the neighbours mainly, because of the neighbours so I just want to go so they [children] don't bother the neighbours and stuff like that.

Like Hassan, Muhammad also faced challenges in maintaining his family's confinement at home during the pandemic. He recounted how the enforced home isolation triggered memories of past traumatic experiences, including civilian curfews and social restrictions resulting from the conflict in Syria and nearby host countries. Muhammad expressed frustration over the lack of consideration for refugees' unique circumstances by neighbours, his children's schoolteachers, and even medical professionals amidst the COVID-19 crisis. While Muhammad acknowledged the necessity of restrictions to ensure his family's safety, he also conveyed the profound difficulty in coping with the confinement. He hopes for a greater understanding of their trauma and experiences from others.

Muhammad's struggle to maintain his children's schooling at home during the pandemic mirrors the challenges faced by other participants. He wanted his kids to have a safe educational and social environment. Other participants shared their difficulties with the transition to online learning. These challenges included feeling unprepared to teach their children, lacking the knowledge of the subjects to teach and the method of instruction, and not having the necessary physical or technological resources to support virtual learning. While the shift to remote classrooms presented challenges for all Canadian families, refugees faced additional obstacles, such as language and technology barriers.

Sarah's experience exemplifies the broader impact of virtual learning and lockdown measures on refugee families. She shared how her son's mental health and ability to cope with daily stressors were affected by the transition to virtual learning. Sarah explained that she could not open the curtains to let natural sunlight into her home, as it caused her son increased anxiety:

> In March COVID happens. We stayed at home since March. Until now my son doesn't even want me to open the curtain to look outside. He's having a severe depression. I cannot get him to go outside or even open the curtain, look through the window, or anything else. So now he's staying at home. He's not going to any school. He is in the house alone and he doesn't even want his own brother to be near him. He doesn't want anybody to be near him. He doesn't want his father. He doesn't want anybody to get near him. He is so depressed. It's so hard to communicate with others online and share the activities with other kids. It is too hard for him.

Hajra, Muhammad, and Halima voiced concerns about their children experiencing significant setbacks in both their physical and social development since the pandemic began. The lockdowns and school closures mainly affected their disabled children, disrupting their established daily routines and cutting off the educational and social support they relied on at school. Before the pandemic, their children received daily academic and social skills assistance from special education teachers and educational assistants. However, these essential services were halted with the onset of lockdowns, leaving parents without the necessary resources to support their children's communication, behavioural, social, and academic needs at home. Parents working from home had to juggle their employment responsibilities with caring for their children during school hours, adding another layer of complexity to the situation.

Additionally, the pandemic led to many critical pediatric disability-related services that children once accessed outside of school being classified as non-essential. As a result, many children were unable to attend in-person therapies or receive much-needed respite support. Muna spoke about her son's struggles during virtual learning, describing how he became frustrated by his inability to keep up with his peers. He had stopped attending his after-school therapies and struggled to cope with the changes. Muna's story underscores the emotional toll that the pandemic-induced disruptions had on children with disabilities and their families, highlighting the profound impact of these circumstances on their overall well-being:

> So, the past 11 months is virtual because of COVID. He is not going good with computer, and it is difficult for him to focus on the screen and be with the other classmates. It's been almost one year. So, his habits and his way of doing his homework is completely different. He can't keep up with his peers. His problem-solving skills is very bad, he is always angry and frustrated. He's not organized, everything is everywhere, and he is always irritated and always screaming and angry.

Halima recounted the difficulty she faced in conveying to her children the reasons behind the imposed restrictions preventing them from attending school or visiting public places like the mall. They did not understand the necessity of such restrictions, and she had difficulty explaining:

> And now in COVID, I always telling him it's closed. It's closed, the mall is closed so he doesn't want to go anywhere else. He asks to go to the Walmart. He likes that. When COVID hit it got so difficult and there was not a space for them to go or something like that. So, they did not go anywhere, and the older kid it's hard for him to do anything. He only wants to do something he likes or wants. When we couldn't go to Walmart or the mall, it was so hard. Before he used to go to his friend, his dad's friends like to go for a couple of hours but that stopped since COVID.

Hassan described the challenge of sharing his cell phone with his children for their online learning tasks and classroom meetings because he did not own a computer or tablet. Despite promises from the school to provide laptops to students in need, the distributed laptops were older used models. They lacked certain features like cameras, putting Hassan's children at risk of further exclusion from virtual classroom activities because their peers could not see them during sessions. Furthermore, virtual learning often lacked essential accessibility features, such as closed captions on YouTube videos shared by teachers, making it difficult for students with hearing difficulties to participate. Despite the inconvenience, Hassan prioritized his children's inclusion in virtual learning, as his smartphone had a small camera, allowing them to participate more fully in their classes. As a result, he could not communicate with his phone or complete any work tasks during school hours. Even while conducting the interviews, several participants, including Sarah, could not use their own devices as their children required them for school.

Marwa highlighted the importance of high-speed internet for virtual learning. The internet connection at her home was inadequate for her children's virtual sessions. Her child often experienced a lag during videos, causing her to miss content. Marwa felt frustrated by the teacher's response whenever her child was disconnected from the virtual platform, which seemed dismissive of her connectivity issues. Previously, she would go to the public library to use the internet, but the libraries were closed during the pandemic. I thought about the unfair expectations teachers and school boards had for parents and caregivers and how it is assumed that all students have the resources to access necessary technology and have the skills and knowledge to navigate that technology. For example, a certain degree of fluency in the English language is also required for virtual learning.

While conducting virtual interviews with participants from home, my children were also engaged in virtual learning. They were mostly independent with their virtual learning and did not require much supervision or support. To make things easier, my daughter's public-school teacher utilized an application that allowed me to communicate directly with her via my smartphone. This application enables parents to read and respond to messages from the teacher throughout the day, providing regular updates through a messaging system. While I appreciated the convenience of this application for monitoring my child's progress, I could not help but notice the assumption that families were equipped for virtual learning. No one inquired about my access to a smartphone or my ability to navigate the application. I was never offered technical support or an alternative communication method, which would have been crucial if I had not owned a smartphone or spoken English fluently. This assumption that everyone has access to required technology exacerbates the isolation experienced by disabled refugee children and their families and impedes their academic progress and social engagement.

Stories of securing rights

The topic of human rights and disability rights frequently emerged in conversations with the storytellers. Despite Canada's commitment to disability rights as discussed in Chapter Four, disability rights for refugees in Canada remain significantly unrealized. Conversations on human rights tend to overlook the economic and living conditions that contribute to the marginalization of disabled refugees. They are pushed into vulnerable social and economic positions, relying on discriminatory welfare practices with limited access to social services. Many participants asserted that disabled individuals in Canada deserve fundamental rights and freedoms, such as the right to obtain services free from discrimination and harmful practices, the right to equitable education, and the right to access rehabilitative services. Before seeking asylum in Canada, all the participants were led to believe that Canada respects the rights of all persons, including disabled refugees, and ensures their inclusion in all aspects of society.

In one conversation, Omar referred to Canada as 'a human rights country'. He said Canada has been able to provide his son with his acute medical care needs but that his rights as a disabled child have been ignored in other vital areas, such as necessary therapies, education with appropriate accommodations, and access to social support. Omar shared that his son received vaccines upon arrival and was treated fairly whenever he had an acute illness, such as an earache. However, his lifelong critical disability needs are not prioritized. Omar believes too much government funding goes into the aesthetics and design of healthcare buildings and not enough into the quality and quantity of healthcare and social services. 'Have you seen the Sick Kids lobby?' he asked, referring to the Hospital for Sick Children in Downtown Toronto. 'It looks better than any mall or hotel we have where I am from, but… we don't need that', he sighed. 'We need services for children with special needs that protect them and actually help them learn and grow.'

Omar emphasized the importance of allocating funds to address pressing issues within the healthcare system. He highlighted the long wait times for health services, the limited time patients spend with doctors and other healthcare professionals, and the high costs associated with therapies, respite services, and adaptive equipment. Omar questioned why the government prioritizes spending on design and marketing instead of covering essential services like therapies, prescription medications, eye care, and dental care. He further illustrated his point by referencing a local community paediatric rehabilitation agency where his son was denied a required stander due to insufficient funding:

> Considering, like when you look at these buildings, all of them, the decor and the wood, everything is so perfect. But really when you go in there, the service is nothing. So well, I think that if they like instead, they provided us with a stander that he can start to stand on. But like I think it's better to provide them with services like that ... I need for my son like speech therapy, physical therapy, and all of that.

Having a stander would significantly benefit Omar's son by improving his strength, range of motion, and endurance. It would enable him to engage more actively in various activities and enhance his independence by providing better access to various spaces in his environment through different positions, such as standing rather than sitting. As an occupational therapist, I recognize the importance of this equipment for Omar's son's overall well-being and development. Omar emphasized how the stander could also serve as a preventive measure, potentially averting further injuries by stretching his son's legs and providing relief from prolonged sitting. He questioned whether healthcare professionals in Canada prioritize preventative approaches to further health complications for disabled children and whether disabled children are perceived as deserving of a better quality of life. Like Omar, Amal's expectations of the treatment of disabled persons in Canada were far from the reality she experienced:

> Coming to Canada was not what I expected. I expected that here in this country specifically that has a top rank in taking care of people, that I would find what I need. But they do not even give the minimum for disabled people.

Amal conveyed her disappointment with Canada and other nations in the Global North, which are often praised for their progressiveness compared to countries in the Middle East. Without labelling it as such, she described othering within the context of Orientalism (discussed in Chapter Four). She expressed how Arabs are viewed as barbaric and backward, and their healthcare systems are referred to as being less civilized. Amal expected Canada to have robust policies safeguarding the rights of disabled persons. Instead, she discovered that disabled persons often find themselves entangled in a system that subtly discriminates against them, leading to their isolation and marginalization:

> Don't we have human rights here? There is a discrimination in the system, but in a hidden way ... in a hidden way that the person who discriminates is not, uh, like is not treated like he's not guilty for what he did, or you cannot see anything to prove that he discriminated.

Amal's comments about human rights are frequently echoed by the families I work with at SMILE Canada. For example, Sana, a Pakistani Muslim mother, shared how her inquiries about her disabled child were consistently disregarded at the local children's hospital by the attending doctor until her white spouse joined her in the examination room. Suddenly, the staff became more friendly, attentive, and forthcoming with information. Like many of the participants, Parents involved with SMILE have reported explicit and implicit discrimination, including Islamophobic, xenophobic, racist, and ableist comments from healthcare providers. The examples are numerous: from healthcare workers questioning whether a disabled youth is oppressed for wearing hijab or questioning whether fasting in Ramadan promotes eating disorders. Too often, healthcare practitioners have dismissed the validity of parents' and caregivers' concerns and knowledge. As Hajra exemplified:

> I get discrimination because I wear hijab and I have had really bad times – and because I don't speak English – not everywhere. There are people who are helpful and really nice, but there are places where I meet people who are rude to me, and I don't know why.

Hajra's experience speaks to a broader climate of exclusion, where cultural and linguistic differences are often met with hostility or ignorance.

Halima shared how her daughter's teacher reported that the coat she wore over her clothes was inappropriate. The teacher said it must make her feel hot and further isolates her from her peers since her disability already makes her stand out in the classroom.

> She used to wear the Syrian coat. Usually, in Syria, they wear a jilbab, a short light coat in the summer on top of their clothes,

and so everyone was telling her why are you doing that way? Wearing that and they kept like saying things about it. So, she just took it off, she started to wear just the shirt and the pants like so. I asked her how she felt, she said, she felt horrible. She said to me, 'I am not from Syria, I am Syria'.

As I listened to Halima's story of Islamophobic and xenophobic encounters at school, I could not help but think about all the harmful questions and comments I received as a young racialized Muslim woman who wore hijab at school: 'Are you hot in this?', 'Are you bald underneath that thing?', 'Do you shower with it on?', 'Do your parents force you to dress that way?' After my conversation with Halima, I reflected on how exhausted I always felt from such inappropriate and offensive questions from peers and teachers. Defending my choices, culture, and faith was an extra exercise many of my peers did not have to do.

Participants stressed the significance of safe spaces. These are places where they are treated with respect and protected from stigma and discrimination. Moreover, they raised the issue of the right to accessible information. This conversation is especially vital for disabled refugees, as essential information is frequently conveyed assuming that patients or clients speak English and have the necessary resources, technology, and knowledge to navigate healthcare systems. Like the challenges faced with virtual platforms during online learning, the technology utilized to navigate the healthcare system assumes one has the technology and understands how to use it.

All participants encountered language barriers when seeking services and support, a common challenge in the resettlement process in Canada (Danso, 2002). Muna, for example, emphasized the necessity of interpretation services at all appointments. She shared how she has never been asked if she requires an interpreter. The responsibility is on her to request interpretation services at every appointment. However, with interpreters unavailable due to COVID-19 protocols, she was compelled to navigate virtual appointments in English. Unfortunately, her doctor's inability to understand her and reluctance to provide clear explanations left Muna disappointed and frustrated. Marwa echoed similar communication struggles, particularly in advocating for her children's needs to teachers. Despite her persistent efforts, teachers failed to translate materials appropriately or simplify content, hindering her ability to effectively support her children's education.

Sarah's experience underscores a troubling reality: despite her right to request an interpreter, healthcare workers often leave her feeling inferior when she does so. Instead of providing professional interpretation services, she is frequently asked to bring a family member despite having no immediate family in Canada besides her children. For Sarah, the challenges of communication are further complicated by her efforts to navigate English and American Sign Language (ASL). Sarah has been learning English to better advocate for her deaf child, but her progress has been hindered by her caregiving responsibilities at home. While her children have been learning ASL to communicate with teachers and peers, Sarah has yet to receive formal instruction in sign language and private ASL classes are expensive. Instead, she has improvised gestures or relied on signs she learned in Syria, where she had limited exposure to a deaf community. She described communicating with her children in the only way she knows:

> I learned sign language by myself to communicate with my children with special needs. My English is not so bad, but I am trying to learn better English so I can talk to the doctors and lawyers and do everything on my own. I want to learn English, but I am stuck because I need also to take care of my children.

Muhammad left me with a critical point of reflection before we ended our conversation. 'Really, what rights do we truly possess?' he asked rhetorically. His question is a powerful reminder of the necessity for systemic reforms that address intersectional oppressions, ensuring that rights of disabled refugees are truly realized in Canada.

Stories of gratitude

All the participants expressed their gratitude for entering Canada at one point or another. They expressed gratitude to the Canadian government for allowing Syrian refugees to settle in Canada. They thanked God for giving them a 'second chance' and the 'Canadian people' for accepting them. Several participants compared themselves to those in Syria who did not or could not seek asylum. While I understand and empathize with their deep sense of relief and appreciation for safety, it prompted me to ask: what expectations of gratitude are instilled through the dominant narrative. This prevailing narrative, which seems to be the only one accepted in public discourse, oversimplifies the refugee experience, particularly in Canada's resettlement context. It glosses over the intricate complexities of transnational experiences and the diverse forms of oppression refugees may encounter in their new environment. There's a common assumption that the challenges refugees face in Canada are trivial compared to the hardships endured in their countries of origin. However, this oversimplification fails to acknowledge the nuanced realities of resettlement, including the social and economic hurdles families face as they navigate unfamiliar systems.

During my conversation with Mohammed, his deep sigh was followed by a heartfelt statement: 'I am very thankful for being in Canada, but …'. This preamble set the stage for his acknowledgement of the lack of support his family receives. Mohammed elaborated on how parents and families are seldom consulted about their children's needs; instead, they are provided with what others assume they require. Similarly, Omar echoed Mohammed's reaction by initially expressing gratitude for being in Canada, then quickly describing the challenges his family faces:

> I handle everything, I am thankful for everything, but I found it difficult, the expenses and the hate. Sometimes when we think of where we've come from and it's really difficult, and then we're trying to, you know, come to be thankful for where we are. But as Muslims we always say we will handle, and we want, you know, to be grateful for whatever we do, whatever we suffer in our lives.

Growing up in a Muslim family, I am intimately familiar with the concept of شكر (shukr), which Omar referenced repeatedly. Shukr is an Arabic term that encapsulates gratitude or thankfulness. Hassan believes Allah (the one God) has given him the capacity to handle whatever challenges come his way, but his concern lies with his disabled children. He desires their belonging and safety and wants them to have the resources not only to survive but also to lead purposeful and meaningful lives. While the notion of gratitude, as understood within the Islamic faith, is deeply ingrained within the Quran and Sunnah (prophetic tradition), and plays a crucial role in shaping one's narrative, it is often co-opted by the dominant cultural narrative in a way that perpetuates otherness and reinforces xenophobic stereotypes. Gratitude, as I comprehend it in my faith, is intertwined with several other Islamic ethical principles, such as justice, dignity, and equity.

While I listened to the stories of gratitude, I could not help but reflect on the settler-colonial dynamics at play. The expressions of gratitude towards Canada seemed to be directed towards white-settler Canadians. Growing up, I, too, was conditioned to believe that we owed a debt of gratitude to 'white' Canada for granting us the freedom to immigrate, live, learn, work, and experience life in Canada. This narrative portrayed Canada's power and heritage solely through the lens of white settlers. I was never taught to thank Indigenous persons for taking up space on this land. Even when land acknowledgements became prevalent in public spaces, the discussions around acknowledging land remained surface level and extremely hypocritcal. They did not lead to further discussions of reparations or realization of Indigenous rights. Expressing gratitude towards white settlers for being allowed into Canada perpetuates a narrative that further marginalizes refugees and reinforces their status as foreigners, hindering their belonging to society. In the same breath, Hajra expressed her love for Canada and her disappointment that disabled children are not being taken care of:

> I do love Canada so much and Canada is like my mother, and I think Canada can do good things but I'm disappointed that kids with special needs are struggling, there has to be some support. All the doctors who aren't helping, someone should talk to them and make them understand that there needs to be more services for special needs kids. They need help.

Thinking back to Hajra's comments about the lack of support for disabled children, I recalled a meeting with an executive director of a health agency to discuss more adequate resources for Sudanese refugees. During this meeting, he proclaimed his envy for refugees upon their arrival in Canada. About refugees being temporarily housed in local hotels, he sarcastically remarked, 'I wish I could stay at a hotel for months'. My heart sank. My experiences visiting these temporary shelters paint a starkly different picture. Far from luxurious, the living conditions were often cramped with rationed resources. I remember encountering a Sudanese family of seven confined to a one-bedroom hotel room with a single, inaccessible bathroom. They waited nearly a year for a settlement worker to assist them in finding a more suitable living situation. Their child lacked access to necessary adaptive equipment and assistive technology throughout their stay, rendering basic activities like bathing unsafe. During my visits to temporary shelters, I witnessed children lined up in long queues to receive food and clothing. Portions were rationed so that one family 'doesn't take too much', according to one of the volunteers at the settlement agency. I witnessed families sifting through piles of used clothing and household items, all while being policed for taking only what they were instructed. I observed silently as caseworkers and volunteers remarked how lucky the families were to receive any supplies at all.

Stories of inclusion

Throughout the discussions, the topic of inclusion surfaced frequently, underscoring participants' profound longing for safe settings where they could belong. They stressed the significance of creating safe spaces where their families could engage fully, whether in classrooms, social settings, recreational activities, or decision-making forums. Additionally, they underscored the harmful repercussions of societal exclusion. For Muna, the acceptance of her child with a disability into school was transformative. It marked a significant milestone in her life, signifying not just access to education but also recognition and acceptance within the broader community:

> They go to school, and they are enjoying, and even my disabled son is going to school, and I am happy that I found a school that could accept him and do activities for him. In Arabic country, nobody will give me any of those services there. Instead, he be like home sleeping, you know, understand what I mean. But, uh, but mostly here it's comfortable.

Other parents' experiences in public school were less positive. Sarah recounted her son's profound loneliness at public school. He struggled to make friends, and teachers seemed only to perceive him through the lens of his disability. When her son became upset at school, his teachers lacked the skills and empathy to address his behaviours. He was often excluded from classroom and school-wide events and activities. For example, while other students attended school assemblies, her son remained behind in the classroom with a teacher. Sarah explained how this exclusion and isolation further upset her son, leading him to express himself through yelling or throwing things. She knew her son's behaviours were not widely accepted at school, but she urged his teachers to consider how the exclusion and isolation further exacerbated problematic behaviours:

> I tried to send him to public school, and he was so lonely. He was so aggressive. He was so aggressive in the bus it didn't work well. Both of my children were accepted into the private schools for kids with special needs. There are private programmes for deaf and blind children.

Sarah described her experience with private schools as 'exceptional', noting that the staff understood her children's needs. However, her children were only accepted to the school for two years and removing them from a place they felt seen and safe was cruel. Her children got accustomed to communicating with experienced teachers working with children with specific accessibility needs. Sarah said that her children are likely to regress significantly, but she has no choice but to send them back to public school. She does not have the financial means necessary to send them to an alternate school.

Halima also faced challenges with her children's schooling in the public system. Concerned about their lack of participation in the classroom, she volunteered at the school for several months to observe their social interactions and advocate for them. During this time, Halima noticed that her disabled children were repeatedly ignored in the classroom. They were given tablets for extended periods, often spending the day playing alone with minimal instruction. The children were seated away from their peers and were not provided with differentiated instruction to meet their needs. When Halima complained about her children being excluded from the classroom, the teacher attributed the lack of classroom support to funding cuts in Ontario under premier Doug Ford's leadership.

Upon hearing this, I was reminded of similar concerns voiced by teachers at my children's public school. A memo issued in February 2021 by Deputy Minister Nancy Naylor highlighted severe cuts to various classroom roles, including mental health workers, early childhood educators, and paraprofessional staff.

These cuts disrupted crucial support provided to disabled children within the school system, threatening their education and future opportunities (Press Progress, 2021). The paradox in the response from teachers around the exclusion of disabled children was that it was attributed to available resources, rather than recognizing their inherent right to equitable education.

Hajra made the difficult decision to transfer her children from public school to a private Islamic school. However, upon enrolment, she discovered that the Islamic school did not offer her children an Individualized Education Plan (IEP) and could not adequately address their diverse needs in learning, sensory processing, physical abilities, behaviours, and social interactions. According to the Ontario Ministry of Education (2018), '[a]n IEP identifies the student's specific learning expectations and outlines how the school will address these expectations through appropriate accommodations, programme modifications and/or alternative programmes as well as specific instructional and assessment strategies'. This identification was necessary for her child to thrive in school. Not only was Hajra paying out of pocket for her child to attend Islamic school, but she also had to pay for a teaching assistant and additional academic resources for him to learn. While she was happy that her children belonged and were respected for their cultural and faith identities, she sacrificed the quality of her son's education. Hajra compared the educational experiences of her non-disabled child and her disabled child. While her non-disabled child is encouraged by teachers to excel academically and develop their social and communication skills, as well as explore potential career paths, her disabled child receives only a minimal standard of education and is often engaged in repetitive, mundane activities:

> I want my child to do well and reach his full potential. Kids are supposed to come first. On the other hand, my daughter [without a disability] has a good teacher, they believe in her, they push her, they believe in her. I came here because this country has rights for people. And kids come first.

Similarly, Muna recounted how her disabled child is often neglected by teachers who prioritize teaching neurotypical students. She explained that while the inclusion model could be beneficial for her child's learning and social skills, it backfires when the teacher fails to attend to the needs of the disabled students in the classroom. Muna further described how the educational system is designed to keep disabled kids feeling lesser than non-disabled kids. Hajra shared this sentiment, rhetorically and sarcastically asking, 'What is so special about special education?'.

We sat in silence for a few moments, reflecting on the weight of these words, before Hajra moved on to discuss how, in addition to being part of a discriminatory education system, her child is further excluded from learning opportunities and social activities within her own faith and cultural community. Her child cannot attend the Sunday religious school or after-school Quran programmes. Community members often stare at her child with pity. Her family is rarely invited to community events or parties or asked to participate in children's programmes. Hajra wants her kids to learn about their culture and faith and interact with others who understand the challenges of migrating to a new place. However, if her disabled child is not included in spaces, then her entire family is excluded.

Throughout the discussions, the storytellers emphasized the significance of feeling accepted, welcomed, and respected in all settings, as well as the importance of forming social relationships. Dalia's story, in particular, illustrates the transformative impact of social relationships in her resettlement journey. Shortly after arriving in Canada, she met Afnaan, a Palestinian woman who became her best friend and most powerful advocate. Afnaan helps Dalia with daily tasks such as buying groceries and scheduling appointments. She also helps Dalia advocate for her needs and facilitates connections with other women who have experienced similar challenges of forced migration and armed conflict. While the support and advocacy are helpful, Dalia emphasized how Afnaan's presence is the most significant source of comfort. She feels safe disclosing her experiences to Afnaan as she, too, endured many obstacles, such as fleeing occupation in Palestine and seeking asylum in Canada, which she believed shaped her compassion towards others. Dalia's experience underscores the crucial role of social connections in navigating the complexities of resettlement and finding support during difficult times.

At SMILE Canada, we emphasize the African proverb 'It Takes a Village', highlighting the crucial role of community support while raising children. This concept of collective responsibility resonates deeply within many cultural communities, including my own. Reflecting on my upbringing, I recognize the privilege of receiving extensive social, emotional, and material support from my extended family and community, as well as having a safe space to share my authentic life stories. Many participants described leaving their 'village of support' of close-knit communities behind in their home country and are now raising their children alone in Canada.

Stories of advocacy

Participants shared their challenges in advocating for their family's intersectional and unique needs. Their narratives demonstrate resilience and determination, as they work tirelessly to ensure their voices are heard. They know their stories the best. They were and are in the best position to advocate for their needs and the needs of their children. Muna's experiences with healthcare workers highlight the need for ongoing advocacy for her disabled son:

> We don't have to pay but there are a lot of difficulties I have been through. It's not like I expected before I came here. I was hoping to find answers. I went here to the children's hospital and was hoping that they do at least like a CT scan for his head because he had meningitis, and they didn't follow up. They told me his head is not like other kids, but they didn't tell me what is wrong with him. They gave him medication to calm him down and to make him less hyperactive. So, they finally did a CT scan eight months ago for him after I kept asking but I don't know the results.

The clinicians' response to Muna's child was to prescribe a mild sedative aimed at reducing his hyperactivity. However, Muna felt that such medications failed to address the underlying cause of the issues he experienced. Beyond his diagnosed developmental disability, he had endured years of physical and emotional trauma related to displacement, poverty, sanctions, and military violence. These medications, in Muna's view, only scratched the surface of the complex challenges her child faced, neglecting the deeper physical, emotional, and psychological impacts of his story. Furthermore, the wait for her child's results is daunting. At that moment in the conversation, I thought about how many local hospitals and clinics advertise web applications like PocketHealth, which, for a monthly fee, allow patients to look up the results of health tests and reports within days of the appointment. While these services are helpful, they are only available to those who can afford the cost and have the digital literacy to navigate the application. Muna, in contrast, continues to wait for a specialist to call her in to discuss her child's results.

Similarly to Muna, Amal shared her challenges in navigating the healthcare system for her disabled child. Not only did she struggle to locate the necessary services, but she also felt uncertain about which services her child actually required. Many recommended therapies were unfamiliar to her. For example, applied behaviour analysis and occupational therapy were underscored as necessary. However, Amal questioned the significance of these services when she had never heard of them before coming to Canada. Listening to her, I recalled a particular statement from the photo essay authored by Church et al. (2020, p. 121): '[d]isabled childhoods are constructed less around individuals' experiences of bodily difference than they are around encounters with professional assessment and diagnostic identification, often beginning at birth'.

Both Muna and Hajra shared concerns about their interactions with Canadian physicians, noting that physicians spent minimal time interacting with their children yet swiftly diagnosed them with lifelong conditions. They both emphasized the impossibility of sharing their complex stories within a brief consultation window where parents can only address one concern at a time. The two storytellers highlighted how doctors relied solely on behavioural checklists and verbal assessments for information gathering. Muna and Hajra were handed standardized forms in English without considering potential language barriers or cultural nuances and were expected to complete them independently. This approach left both of them feeling unheard and frustrated, as their children's unique needs and circumstances were overlooked in favour of standardized procedures. Muna shared:

> This is not fair for my son and not fair for me as I don't know what to do with him or where to take him. The doctors who diagnose autism should be in the know of the services that we can seek or what funds we can apply to. We are only allowed to give them one issue when we go to the doctor. If we tell them what is happening with us, they tell us that it is not the

> time to speak about those things. Even the doctor took all the things he needs to know from me as a parent, not from him [child with a disability]. The doctor does not even know what he can do or anything.

Hajra was overwhelmed by the level of support her child required to improve his academic and social skills. Expressing her inability to fulfil multiple roles, such as that of a mother, teacher, therapist, and nurse, she found it deeply unfair to be expected to juggle all these responsibilities alone. While searching for help, Hajra came across a Kumon office one day while walking in her neighbourhood. Kumon is an academic tutoring service known for its success in improving children's math and reading abilities. Despite the classes being expensive, Hajra was determined to support her child's learning and enrolled him in weekly afterschool Kumon classes, paying for them privately. She exhausted her disability support funds at Kumon on a tutor who lacked specialized training to work with children with disabilities:

> I am very sad that I couldn't find anybody to show us where to go to get resources or help for him. And the thing that didn't help, I used all my money for Kumon and for tutors. And they wouldn't help him. I didn't know he needs specialized people like occupational therapy and services like that.

During my master's in occupational therapy, I was taught a fundamental principle: the patient or client and, by extension, their family are the true experts in their own story. They know how they feel and can identify the intricacies of their condition or concerns. For example, they can articulate their pain levels, pinpoint where it hurts, and describe the nature of the pain. They understand how these factors affect their daily lives because they live through these experiences. While I may have grasped these concepts in the classroom, my clinical experiences have helped me understand that simply learning about client-centred and family-centred approaches does not always lead to equitable practices being put into action. We must actively and intentionally listen to client narratives. We must believe them and prioritize them.

Client and family-centred care should involve culturally responsive, relevant, and safe methods where families feel included and respected. It should entail an anti-oppressive approach, but it does not. Unfortunately, as Whalley Hammell (2015) points out, there is a need for further critical examination to assess whether healthcare professionals, such as occupational therapists, truly consider their clients' narratives. In my conversation with Hajra, she brought attention to the tendency of healthcare workers to approach patients with a predetermined agenda. When faced with similar diagnoses or conditions, clinicians tend to respond similarly, disregarding individuals' unique and authentic stories. For Hajra, it was perplexing how a lifelong diagnosis of attention deficit hyperactivity disorder (ADHD) and autism could be reached within just 15 minutes of meeting with a doctor. I too wondered how a doctor could understand someone's transnational story of disablement during such a short period.

Muna's story also underscores the profound impact of the erasure of authentic patient narratives. She recounted chemical attacks in her hometown in Syria and the devastating impacts these attacks had on civilian populations, including her own family. Upon arriving in Canada, she found that healthcare professionals largely dismissed the significance of these horrific lifechanging events. Muna shared how the doctors and therapists in Canada did not address the danger of chemical weapons her family was exposed to, no matter how much she told them about it. Some physicians she met believed it was irrelevant, while others questioned whether she was telling the truth. The doctors instead only discussed the diagnoses of ADHD and autism. One doctor even prescribed medication that proved harmful, causing her son to become lethargic during the day, rather than addressing his attention issues in school. Muna was deeply concerned that her son was not himself. He seemed tired and distant all the time. Muna continued to seek out medical help for her son, grappling with the emotional toll of the war's lasting effects on his physical and psychological well-being.

Furthermore, Muna expressed frustration at her limited English proficiency, which hinders her ability to advocate effectively for her son in Canada. During our interview, she tearfully recounted an encounter with a doctor who emphasized her son's missed developmental milestones, lecturing her about the importance of early intervention after she shared his experiences with chemical warfare. She reported feeling unjustly punished for circumstances beyond her control, having recently arrived in the country and facing significant challenges navigating its healthcare system. Wiping her tears, she said:

> I took him to another doctor, and the doctor blamed me a lot, and the doctor said you should have helped him in the other years. And me not knowing English is not my problem because if any of you moved to another country, it is not my fault, if you moved to another country, you won't be able to understand what they are saying.

When she visited the second doctor, Muna described how the doctor never once interacted with her child directly. He never looked right at him, shook his hand, asked how he felt or attempted to build trust with him. He also never observed him doing specific tasks or movements to gain his level of skills.

> He asks a couple of questions and that is it. I was imagining that they would talk to him, ask him how he's doing. He only did an assessment one time and then forgot about it.

Some families reported needing the prescribed therapeutic services, such as physical therapy and speech and language therapy. In contrast, others were not interested in the recommended treatments. 'Therapy. Therapy and more therapy. Not everyone wants it or needs it', Hajra shared. Several other participants echoed this sentiment as they discussed the recommendations given to them.

It was this very reflection that led me to pursue a PhD in Critical Disability Studies after several years of practicing as a therapist. I aimed to challenge the notion that therapy alone can 'fix' issues stemming from a disabling oppressive system. I recognized that disabled refugees were not being heard or treated with equity and dignity. They were frequently offered support and resources that may not align with their actual needs.

Muna reported that neither her child's history during the war nor her family history was ever considered during her initial conversation with her child's doctor. The doctor ignored her account of her child's medical and social history and began his story in Canada. While the doctor used terms such as global developmental delay (GDD) and attention deficit hyperactivity disorder (ADHD), she was more concerned about her child contracting meningitis and not getting treated for it:

> I am having difficulty with his diagnosis. I am hoping that I find someone who knows more about his case about the history because everything they give my child is for GDD and I want to know about other things like meningitis. No one [doctors] talks to me about it. I always tried to say to the doctors that his … my son's story starts from the beginning, but they always do not focus on that area and they don't want to listen. They just look at his behaviours and tell me about GDD and ADHD and they take a picture of it at the moment we came here to Canada. Well, every agency here refers them to behavioural therapy, and I don't see any progress.

'Does he need more behaviour therapy'? she said sharply. The behaviour therapy did not yield any results, but therapists continued to prescribe it. There were no noticeable improvements or positive changes in Muna's child's life. She observed that her child played on the iPad during therapy sessions instead of learning how to communicate effectively with others:

> The therapy doesn't suit his case, like he wants to play on his iPad. They tried to tell him how to move to something else, but it doesn't work for him.

Hajra revealed that the therapy recommended for her child not only proved ineffective but also caused harm. Despite her child's resistance to attending therapy sessions, she felt pressured to continue sending him because therapists and caseworkers insisted it was necessary. They even hinted that she would be neglecting her child if she did not comply. Hajra emphasized that she understands her child's needs better than anyone, considering what he has experienced and his reluctance to engage in new activities. Adjusting to numerous unfamiliar social and environmental factors in Canada was already challenging, and the prospect of trying an unfamiliar therapy added to their anxiety. Hajra said, 'But after treatment, he got much, much worse. This is the worst thing they did to him'.

I reflected on Hajra's words in the context of dominant narratives. How was her story being rewritten by people who believed they knew it better than she does? How are they ignoring the intersectional experiences and oppressions that shape her reality? What is the impact of ignoring her story?

Unlike many of the healthcare workers and educators I have worked with over the years, Sarah recognized the significance of discussing disability within the broader context of social determinants of health and disability. Her perspective further underscores the limitations of relying solely on clinical interventions and therapies to support disabled persons and their families. She emphasized the importance of holistic support, including assistance with employment to achieve financial independence rather than reliance on charity and social services. Sarah's insights resonated deeply with me, highlighting her nuanced understanding of transnational disablement. She said:

> I need help with finding support for rent, like the governmental support for a house, like to help me in the rent and seriously for a job for my elder kid. My son, he is finding difficulties finding a job because he's deaf. Nobody accepts him for any job and it's affecting him, and it would be really helpful to find a job. For my other son, I cannot go to work because he needs me all the time. I cannot even leave for five minutes.

Sarah described how a day does not go by without her advocating fiercely for her children. Like Sarah, Hajra also shared how advocacy is vital to her family's survival. She explained how her child is the motive behind her advocacy and how it is her duty to speak up for him; otherwise, he is often disrespected and mistreated. She described how creative and talented her son is at building structures with blocks. 'I can send you pictures', she beamed. Her smile quickly disappeared as she recalled sharing his talent with a doctor, only to have him laugh while watching her son stim with his hands. How could the doctor dismiss her remarks about her son? Hajra did not feel safe in that moment. She came to the appointment seeking help, support, and understanding, but instead, she was met with indifference and a lack of empathy. The doctor's reaction compounded her already growing sense of isolation. How could she trust someone who did not even take the time to listen or acknowledge her child as a person, let alone a person with unique abilities and needs? She felt that her concerns were trivialized and her role and expertise as a mother was belittled.

CHAPTER 6
Listening to our stories

While each participant shared their story, I knew it was only a tiny piece of a much larger puzzle of genuine interwoven transnational narratives. I listened intentionally, absorbing their words, sighs, smiles, and tears. I noticed the subtle changes in their tones as they recounted being forcibly displaced from their homes, leaving everything they knew behind. I heard the tremble in their voices as they spoke about the immense loss of human life and the fear of losing family members and friends. Amidst the heartache, I also sensed their relief and optimism when they spoke of their children's safety in Canada and aspirations for their children's future. This exercise of actively listening and reflecting was undertaken with careful deliberation, a practice that is critical but not mandatory for doctors, teachers, settlement workers, and anyone working with disabled refugees.

The contents of this book demonstrate that ignoring non-dominant stories has detrimental consequences. Several participants shared how Canadian healthcare and educational professionals failed to acknowledge their unique experiences, attributing them solely to past conflicts. For some, this dismissal manifested in overlooking their current struggles in Canada, urging them to move beyond years of trauma and oppression. Hajra, for example, articulates the need for fair treatment for her child in the classroom without erasing his cultural identity or past experiences. She further stresses the need for a comprehensive assessment of her child's learning requirements and for teachers to implement personalized strategies rather than solely attributing his difficulties to the war and neglecting to address his current educational, physical, and social needs:

> I sent him to school, and everyone (teacher and principal) labelled that everything that was wrong with him was due to the war in Syria.

For many participants, having their stories of war, structural violence, and displacement validated was essential. However, they often encountered dismissive attitudes, suggesting they were exaggerating or overreacting to their circumstances. Furthermore, participants expressed frustration that their children's health conditions were frequently questioned or discounted due to a perceived lack of 'appropriate' or 'valid' medical records from their home countries. As a result, they faced significant delays in accessing support services, enduring lengthy waits for appointments and resorting to costly private assessments. The idea that Western, Global North healthcare is inherently superior to Global South healthcare is one embedded within dominant narratives surrounding disabled refugees. In this context, parents' perspectives on their child's condition are typically dismissed unless they are confirmed by Canadian healthcare providers. For example, Muna pleaded with doctors to consider the long-term effects of meningitis on her child, rather than focusing exclusively on developmental disabilities, but her concerns were ignored.

A family-centred approach appeared relevant only when professionals agreed with the family's perspective. As someone who helped refugees navigate healthcare services and discussions around diagnoses, Naima repeatedly saw diagnoses from other countries disregarded, with some professionals even displaying disdain or scepticism towards parents' descriptions or explanations of their child's disability or condition. For Naima, the issue goes beyond simply listening to patient and family narratives; it encompasses a more profound need for acknowledgement and respect:

> I think it ... it's not so much listening to their parents. It's something even bigger. It's about the non-Canadian to Canadian process. Canadians feel the way or system here is superior to the so-called third world. We discount everything that is shared with us based on the idea that our knowledge is superior.

Like Naima, Najma also heard numerous xenophobic comments while accompanying Syrian refugees to medical appointments. These encounters perpetuated the notion that Canadian healthcare was inherently superior to healthcare in Syria and surrounding areas. This belief had dangerous consequences, implying that the participants did not understand their health experiences or the health experiences of their children. For example, Hassan was taken aback when a Canadian doctor informed him, in an insensitive way, that, for years, his children had been completely misdiagnosed.

The doctor spoke about a disease that Hassan had never heard of before. Hassan was filled with guilt and had no time to process the information or question why previous doctors had provided different diagnoses and explanations for his children's conditions. Furthermore, the Canadian doctor presented the information in a manner devoid of empathy, failing to consider Hassan's prior experiences or the reasons behind the differing diagnoses. Instead, they offered an overly simplified explanation, attributing the misdiagnosis to the previous physicians' lack of medical knowledge. A culturally safe and family-centred approach involves establishing and nurturing trust with clients. However, the Canadian doctor's approach resulted in feelings of hurt and mistrust.

Muna shares her experience of a doctor not allowing her the opportunity to discuss her son's trauma, showing little interest in understanding her child's background before they arrived in Canada. Despite Muna's attempts to convey years of extreme poverty and displacement, as well as current housing and food insecurities and ongoing physical and emotional violence, the doctor swiftly asserted his professional authority. He emphasized that he could conduct his diagnostic assessment using the tools and information available. Dismissing Muna's concerns, he also reminded her that his medical office was reserved for one medical issue per visit. As highlighted in the 'Stories of advocacy' section, several participants found their narratives dismissed and overshadowed. Their stories underscore the importance of service providers actively listening to patients' or clients' stories with care and attention, even if it means addressing multiple, connected issues in a single visit.

During these discussions, I kept thinking back to a book I read a few years ago, titled *The social transformation of American medicine*, by Paul Starr (1982). Starr provides a historical overview of the American medical system's development, highlighting the rise of physicians as a social class and exploring the roots of their lasting power. Reflecting on the conversation with Muna, I found Starr's insights remarkably pertinent. Starr discusses how medical professionals have become the gatekeepers of healthcare, with their professional expertise often overshadowing other vital perspectives, particularly those of patients and their families. None of the participants expressed a desire to exclude physicians from their stories; instead, they wanted to be heard by them. The dismissive and authoritative attitude displayed by Muna's physician was not only culturally insensitive but also harmful to her family. Just as the history of American medical culture has tended to view disability as solely a health issue requiring medical intervention, rather than recognizing society's responsibility to address systemic barriers, it has also overlooked the intersectional factors such as disablement and displacement that profoundly affect an individual's health and well-being.

Amal recounts how ignoring her story led to a devastating, life-altering personal tragedy. Several months before our interview, Amal became pregnant with her third child. Having previously had two healthy pregnancies where she carried her children to term, Amal was no stranger to the pregnancy process. However, during the final trimester of her third pregnancy, Amal began experiencing significant pain and excessive bleeding – clear signals that something was wrong with her baby. Despite her stated distress and repeated attempts to express her concerns to the nurses and doctors at the hospital, they consistently dismissed her symptoms. They refused her requests for a thorough physical examination. One nurse said that Amal might be experiencing pain due to sitting in her wheelchair for long periods. She told the nurse that this pain was nothing like anything she had experienced in the past and reassured the nurse that she knew the difference. During our conversation, Amal shared how it was not language or environmental barriers that harmed her: it was a blatant disregard for her narrative. Holding back tears, she rhetorically asks if it is because she is Muslim and wears a hijab, is an Arab, is a refugee, or if it is because she is disabled:

> When I went to get medical care from the emergency, I was pregnant in the third trimester. I had bleeding and cramps, and I asked the doctor to test me. But the doctor was asking why I came to the emergency, he kept saying to go to my family doctor, but I said I didn't have one. The doctor said it's normal and I can go home. I was giving the doctor options; I asked them, why don't you do an ultrasound? I asked if they need to do any blood work or anything? He said no, nothing. I was so scared, then he told me to follow up with my family doctor, but I kept saying I don't have one. But he sent me home. I went home. After five or six hours, I lost my baby.

Amal shares how her comfort lies in the belief that the loss of her child is ultimately in the hands of Allah, but she strongly asserts that doctors must do everything in their power to assist their patients. Despite her urgent need for medical attention, the emergency doctor insisted that Amal visit her family doctor. Amal reiterated that she did not have one, yet the healthcare team disregarded her comments and pleas for help. Amal further explained to the emergency hospital staff how she had recently relocated to the city and lacked the necessary support network. Compounding the challenge was her requirement for wheelchair-accessible facilities and language interpretation services, which were not readily available. Amal's experience reflects the systemic barriers faced by disabled refugees within the healthcare system. When she rushed to the emergency room seeking medical attention for her unborn child, she was sent away without a full assessment, including essential medical tests. As a disabled refugee, Amal felt betrayed by the same healthcare system that vowed to protect her. Ignoring her story had a devastating outcome.

During the interview, I could not fully empathize with Amal's heartbreaking account of losing her child. However, roughly six months later, I experienced a similar tragedy when I laid my own prematurely born baby, Aasiyah, to rest. Reflecting on that painful time, I vividly remember a moment when the anaesthesiologist rushed into my hospital room unexpectedly to administer an epidural for pain management. I grabbed my hijab to cover my hair. He barely paused and ignored the butterfly on the door, which indicates the loss of a child. As he started pulling the giant needle into my spine, he quickly asked if there were any complications he should be aware of. With tears streaming down my face, I yelped, 'Yes, my baby died'. I was exhausted, emotional, and taken aback by his insensitive tone, but what he said next felt like a sharp blow to an open wound. Instead of acknowledging my grief, he callously remarked, 'It's been a busy day. Do you know how many of these I've had to do?' I yelled for him to get out of the hospital room. I would rather experience the pain than have an epidural. The doctor was not listening. He did not hear the fear in my voice, nor did he see the pain in my eyes. He did not respect my cultural or faith traditions. I felt unsafe. His lack of empathy and disregard for my story left a lasting impact, reminding me of the importance of compassion and understanding, especially in moments of profound grief.

As I reflect on my own experience, I am reminded that listening extends beyond mere acknowledgement; it necessitates a deep engagement with the lived experiences of others, rooted in empathy and understanding. It also empowers us to challenge dominant narratives that perpetuate harmful stereotypes and marginalize certain voices. By actively listening to diverse perspectives and embracing non-dominant narratives, we can take responsibility in shaping a more compassionate and inclusive society where every individual's story is heard, respected, and valued. Failing to acknowledge, recognize, and genuinely listen to these stories of disablement and displacement results in partial reception, with detrimental consequences.

As highlighted in Chapter Three, meaningful reflexivity is an essential tool to carefully unpack the dominant narrative that influences research, especially when studying marginalized or underserved populations. While I maintain transparency regarding my various roles as a researcher, healthcare worker, advocate, community organizer, and a Muslim woman of colour, it is important to acknowledge how these roles shape my research process. Reflexivity entails a commitment to actively listen to participants and genuinely engage with their narratives. By allowing ourselves to be vulnerable and embrace discomfort throughout the research journey, reflexivity enables us to confront our assumptions and biases as researchers (Pillow, 2003).

Moreover, framing the discussion around disablement and displacement as a critical issue forces us to recognize the complexity of the problem and its broader implications. While this approach may appear simplistic, acknowledging a situation as problematic opens avenues for potential solutions. Without recognizing the existence of a social health crisis, our sense of urgency to examine the under-served and under-represented positions of disabled refugees globally may diminish.

Advocacy to action

Examining the policies and practices surrounding asylum seeking for disabled displaced persons in Canada and across the Global North is crucial. During the interviews, I heard first-hand accounts of the diverse pathways through which refugees arrive in Canada. Notably, private sponsorship often places the burden of responsibility on families and community members instead of the government. However, there is ambiguity regarding who is accountable for supporting disabled refugees upon their arrival in Canada. Some participants recounted being left to navigate the challenges independently, while others described receiving initial support from private sponsors that dwindled over time. This discrepancy in support raises critical questions: what obligations does Canada have in assisting displaced, disabled individuals? What role should settlement agencies play in supporting disabled children and their families? Upon arrival, families often face barriers in accessing disability-related services such as therapies, adaptive equipment, and assistive technology. They must start from scratch: finding a primary care physician, obtaining referrals to healthcare and disability specialists, and joining funding waitlists. Families arriving in Canada with limited support and resources must shoulder the full responsibility of covering the costs of private disability-related services. Whose job is it to inform newcomers of disability-related services and ensure they can successfully navigate the many social systems? Clarifying these responsibilities is essential as a first step to ensure that disabled refugees receive the support and resources they need to thrive in their new environment.

While these practical challenges highlight the immediate and urgent needs of disabled refugees, they also point to broader systemic issues. Despite significant strides made in advancing Equity, Diversity, and Inclusion (EDI) initiatives across Canada (Ramirez, 2021)—including policies on truth and reconciliation, systemic discrimination, and examining internal biases and privileges, a notable gap persists in addressing disability and ableism within these dialogues. Frequently, discussions result in an EDI checklist of identities that overlooks the intersectional experiences of oppression encountered by disabled persons, particularly refugees and newcomers who navigate the intricate interplay between national and transnational narratives.

The narratives shared by participants in this study reveal that disabled refugees face a multitude of environmental and attitudinal obstacles, as well as exclusionary practices, in their daily lives. These challenges highlight the need for inclusive and culturally safe health and wellness support that acknowledges their unique experiences, which include transnational stories of displacement and disablement. Culturally safe practice involves culturally responsive, relevant, and appropriate resources and services (Williams, 2023). Moreover, participants' narratives also underscore the urgent need for a critical examination of ableist policies and practices that disproportionately affect racialized communities, such as the Syrian newcomer community.

Despite the increasing recognition of the complexity of intersectional identities within EDI frameworks, current service delivery models often fail to address the diverse and critical needs of disabled refugees and their families. This results in a lack of holistic, culturally safe care that fails to adequately address their needs. Existing diagnostic and health assessment frameworks in the Global North overlook the importance of narrative sharing, particularly transnational narratives, unless intentional individual efforts are made to incorporate them. During health assessments, inquiries typically revolve around the medical history of conditions such as one's history of high blood pressure or heart disease, but seldom do they delve into conversations regarding the many social determinants of health and disability that significantly impact the lives of disabled refugees, such as poverty, housing, or food security. Furthermore, it is unclear who is responsible for advocating for the patient once they disclose such information to healthcare providers. For instance, if a patient or client reports insufficient access to food, is there a federal or provincial mandate to refer them to appropriate resources, or are such considerations omitted from health discussions? In the case of disabled refugees, it becomes crucial to listen to stories of trauma-physical and psychological, as well as intergenerational and transnational. The participants' stories reveal that discussions about trauma, displacement, and even exposure to chemical warfare are systemically overlooked.

Incorporating critical aspects of culturally safe support into healthcare assessments and service delivery models can better address the multifaceted needs of disabled refugees, while also fostering a more inclusive and supportive society. Achieving culturally responsive healthcare demands a comprehensive strategy that involves improving the education and training of service providers to deepen their understanding of various experiences and forms of oppression. This training should commence during students' education, before they enter the workforce, with the understanding that culturally responsive care is not an optional addition but essential for ensuring the safety and well-being of clients and patients.

Moreover, addressing entrenched power imbalances and personal biases within the Canadian healthcare system is crucial. Policymakers must engage in a critical evaluation of their cultural privileges that benefit from a dominant narrative and (at minimum) acknowledge the systemic impact of Canada's colonial and settler-colonial history on organizational structures, including hospitals and children's rehabilitation services. Training in culturally safe practices and increasing organizational awareness of equity frameworks are vital steps in this process, but not without addressing past and present settler-colonial ideologies, policies, and ongoing harmful practices. This endeavour requires adopting anti-oppressive, anti-xenophobic, anti-racist, anti-ableist, anti-Islamophobic, and trauma-informed approaches. By integrating these components of culturally responsive support, we can create safer, more inclusive environments for disabled refugees, providing services they need and desire rather than imposing those they may not want or require.

CHAPTER 7
Final reflections

As I conclude this book, three years after the initial phase of my research, I am deeply troubled by the ongoing separation of displacement, structural violence, and intersectional oppressions from vital conversations about health, disability, and human rights. While the number of refugees has increased globally over the past decade (Donato and Ferris, 2020), the experiences of disabled refugees and their families continue to be understudied (Mirza, 2011) and ignored (Crock et al., 2012; Pisani and Grech, 2015). In this final reflection, I critically ask: where are the authentic stories of disabled refugees? How has the segregation of disablement and displacement impacted disabled refugees and their families in the Global North? Why are these profound intersections overlooked in critical conversations on human rights, social justice, and social determinants of health and disability?

Throughout this book, I underscore the power of storytelling – both the content of stories and the experiences they convey. I highlight the grave danger of perpetuating a dominant narrative that fails to capture the complexity of human experiences (Adichie, 2009) and, specifically, the collective patterns of oppression experienced by disabled refugees. Despite the growing recognition of storytelling in research, a settler-colonial tactic of questioning the authenticity and validity of human stories persists, thereby perpetuating the dominant narrative that tells their stories for them.

This is evident in Canada's response to the Syrian refugee crisis. Within this discourse, Canada is deemed heroic, a saviour to Syrian refugees through 'Operation Syria'. This hero narrative is accompanied by the gratitude narrative – disabled Syrian refugees should be thankful for the opportunity to live and be protected. Through this portrayal, disabled refugees are rendered helpless, dependent, and indebted to 'white' Canadians. The stories shared in this text highlight how this gratitude narrative, which may not seem explicitly harmful, reinforces an expected level of assimilation into Canadian culture (Scott and Safdar, 2017). This narrative bleeds into policies and practices tied into Islamophobic, xenophobic, racist, and ableist tropes that implicitly and explicitly make the concept of full citizenship impossible for disabled refugees. When Halima's daughter was asked by her teacher to remove her jilbab to fit in with her classmates, she could not belong as she was. She became othered by her disability, her faith, and her culture. Removing her garment did not make her fit in with the rest of her peers; it further isolated her. As a young child, she recognized that as a disabled Syrian refugee, she could not exist as is. Her story had to be rewritten.

I have come to realize that narrative research, in its potential to unveil lived realities, has the power to help us unlearn and relearn. Through the detailed and personal accounts provided by the storytellers, a narrative qualitative approach allows for a deeper and more empathetic engagement with stories. It helps to uncover systemic issues and barriers that may not be visible through traditional research methods, providing a richer and more comprehensive picture of real storied lives. Furthermore, by documenting and sharing these narratives, this study aims to influence policy and practices around disabled refugees. It seeks to inform policymakers, practitioners, and the broader public about the specific requirements and rights of disabled refugees. This heightened awareness can serve as a catalyst for necessary social and systemic change.

We must not overlook or diminish the realness of human experiences. It is time to move beyond the quantitative data that focuses solely on the number of disabled refugees admitted into Canada, and instead centre the narratives that address their intersectional needs and lived experiences. By prioritizing the stories of Marwa, Amal, Halima, Muhammad, Hajra, Hassan, Muna, Sarah, Omar, Dalia, and their families, we acknowledge the significance of their unique histories and experiences. Their struggles, challenges, and oppressions cannot be dismissed or silenced. Instead, they must be listened to, understood, and ultimately valued.

The 11 major themes presented in this book are not meant to be exhaustive. We must persist in exploring other authentic, non-dominant narratives of disabled refugees. A continued exploration enables us to glean insights from genuine experiences and to challenge and overcome biases inherent in our traditional teachings and understanding. Future examination of the theoretical perspectives on critical concepts such as disablement, citizenship, and otherness will also offer us valuable insights into the marginalized position of disabled refugees in Canada and globally. The participants' stories underscore the significance of exploring the transnational dimension of disability. Specifically, engaging a transnational disability theoretical lens allows us to delve into and better appreciate the lived experiences of disabled refugees, as elucidated through their narratives. Muna and Omar vividly describe the direct impacts of international conflict on their children's health conditions, including the scarcity of medical equipment due to sanctions imposed by countries in the Global North. Similarly, Muna and Sarah highlight how the repercussions of war extend to various facets of their family's well-being, such as economic hardship, psychological trauma, limited educational opportunities, and challenges in finding meaningful employment, further compounded by a lack of safety and security.

Such exploration contributes to the existing body of research on disablement and displacement in critical disability studies, while also enriching other academic fields, including social sciences, migration studies, healthcare, and law. Future research should aim to generate more storied content, providing opportunities for disabled displaced persons to share their narratives safely and authentically and contribute to the collective understanding of their lived experiences. The objective of describing the accounts in detail is to elevate participants' stories as the principal narratives. As Barghouti warns, we must resist the tendency to make human stories secondary (Adichie, 2009). The first-person accounts shared in this book challenge us to listen to, reflect on, trust, and share stories of those whose stories (truths) have too often been appropriated.

The disablement of Gaza

This exploration of the lived experiences of displaced disabled individuals is especially urgent as we witness the mass displacement, ongoing violence and systemic disablement in Gaza, where the intersection of displacement and disablement are not just theoretical ideas but daily lived realities. We are living in a time when the stories of people drastically affected by oppressive systems, such as apartheid, occupation, and ethnic cleansing, are being blatantly disregarded. What deeply troubles me is the international community's indifference to the disability crisis in Gaza, which highlights the urgent need to rethink how we understand disability in transnational contexts. Specifically, in the Global North, we witness healthcare institutions, disability agencies, and paediatric forums championing discourse on health and human rights ignore the ongoing genocide and mass disablement of Palestinians. In sifting through the appalling stories of hospitals leveled, schools destroyed and images of the torture, trauma, and maiming of children, I came across a social media post stating, 'Everyone in Gaza is disabled'.

A year has passed, and over 40,000 civilians have been killed, more than 90,000 injured and 10,000 more missing under the rubble (Al Jazeera, 2024). Gaza has seen more persons become disabled from military-grade weapons than any other conflict in recent human history, with an average of 10 children losing at least one limb per day in the past six months of this writing (United Nations, 2024). More children have been killed in Gaza in recent months than in total global conflicts in the last four years (United Nations, 2023), with over 17,000 children orphaned, unaccompanied, or separated (United Nations, 2023). Gaza is considered the most dangerous place to live, especially for children and disabled persons. Yet the dominant narrative echoed in mainstream media rooms reduces Palestinians to collateral damage, unworthy of basic freedoms and protection. This narrative, which ignores disablement within the context of Palestine, dehumanizes and degrades Palestinians, portraying them as subhuman, non-human, and even likening them to animals, thus denying them the most basic and fundamental human rights (Kasraoui, 2023).

This past year, I have witnessed firsthand the silencing of authentic, transnational human stories of displacement and disablement—stories like that of a six-year-old child who fled Gaza with their family in search of refuge in Canada. The child, showing signs of post-traumatic distress, experienced regression in physical and communication skills, exhibited clear signs of trauma, and malnutrition due to the deprivation of food, and water. The child had also been exposed to white phosphorus, a chemical agent with devastating long-term health effects (Khafaei, 2024). However, when the mother presented the child's situation to a Canadian doctor, her concerns were dismissed with the response, "Well, now you are in Canada." The doctor then proceeded to complete an autism checklist without addressing the family's trauma or the profound impact of their experiences. By disregarding the child's story of forced starvation, displacement, and exposure to chemical weapons, the serious effects of transnational disablement and displacement are neglected, which can have devastating consequences for the child's health and well-being as well as for their family, a shattering experience illustrated by the storytellers in this study.

This dismissive response reflects the pervasive dominance of narratives that marginalize the experiences of displaced and traumatized individuals. Yet, despite the prevalence of these dominant narratives, alternative, non-dominant human stories continue to challenge them. With technological advancements and the rise of social media, we have seen these non-dominant narratives of Palestinians shared widely in the most unfiltered, graphic, harrowing ways for the world to witness. These raw human stories, broadcast live, paint a stark picture of both suffering and resilience in the face of unimaginable adversity. Stories of families pulled out of the rubble in pieces, children having their limbs amputated without medicine or anaesthesia, mothers delivering babies in unsanitary conditions, and critically ill, disabled, and vulnerable persons disconnected from life-saving devices as electricity and fuel were cut off to civilian populations (United Nations, 2023). In this digital age, storytelling has evolved from a method of sharing information to a lifeline—a means of protection and protest for those whose voices have long been silenced. What was once a medium for entertainment is now a powerful tool for advocacy, as these stories reach millions of people across public platforms, reshared and amplified worldwide.

While the concept of transnational disablement may not yet be widely recognized, there is a growing awareness of the profound impact of disability within oppressive systems of domination. As I bring this final chapter to a close, I can only reiterate how crucial it is to recognize how privileging dominant narratives and overshadowing non-dominant stories perpetuates the segregation of displacement and disablement, which explicitly harms disabled newcomers. Through this book, I have intended to shed light on the genuine experiences of disablement and displacement as narrated by the participants. It is my sincere hope that this work will provoke critical discussions and advocate for necessary changes that lead to a more inclusive, equitable, and just society for disabled refugees and their families. Their stories matter.

References

Adichie, C. (2009). The danger of a single story. [Video]. TED. https://www.ted.com/talks/chimamanda_ngozi_adichie_the_danger_of_a_single_story

Ahmed, S. (2017). Trump halts refugee program; Trudeau tweets they're welcome in Canada. CNN, 29 January. https://www.cnn.com/2017/01/29/politics/justin-trudeau-refugees-welcome-trnd/index.html

Albanese, F. (2024, March 24). *Anatomy of a genocide: Report of the Special Rapporteur on the situation of human rights in the Palestinian territory occupied since 1967 to the Human Rights Council – Advance unedited version* (A/HRC/55/73). Human Rights Council. https://www.un.org/unispal/document/anatomy-of-a-genocide-report-of-the-special-rapporteur-on-the-situation-of-human-rights-in-the-palestinian-territory-occupied-since-1967-to-human-rights-council-advance-unedited-version-a-hrc-55/

Aldiabat, K., Alsrayheen, E., Aquino-Russell, C., Clinton, M., & Russell, R. (2021). The lived experience of Syrian refugees in Canada: A phenomenological study. *The Qualitative Report, 26*(2), 484–506. https://doi.org/10.46743/2160-3715/2021.4334

Al Jazeera (2021). Motivated by hate: Muslim family run over in Canada. 7 June. https://www.aljazeera.com/news/2021/6/7/canada-family-targeted-in-fatal-anti-muslim-attack-police-say

Al Jazeera (2024). Israel–Gaza war in maps and charts: Live tracker. https://www.aljazeera.com/news/longform/2023/10/9/israel-hamas-war-in-maps-and-charts-live-tracker

Amnesty International (2023). Israel OPT: US veto of ceasefire resolution displays callous disregard for civilian suffering in face of staggering death toll. 8 December. https://www.amnesty.org/en/latest/news/2023/12/israel-opt-us-veto-of-ceasefire-resolution-displays-callous-disregard-for-civilian-suffering-in-face-of-staggering-death-toll/

Andrews, M., Squire, C., & Tamboukou, M. (Eds.) (2008). *Doing narrative research*. SAGE Publishing.

Angus Reid Institute (2015). *Religion and faith in Canada today: Strong belief, ambivalence and rejection define our views*. 26 March. https://angusreid.org/wp-content/uploads/2016/01/2015.03.25_Faith.pdf

Anthias, F. (2012). Transnational mobilities, migration research and intersectionality: Towards a translocational frame. *Nordic Journal of Migration Research*, *2*(2), 102–110. https://doi.org/10.2478/v10202-011-0032-y

Armenski, T., Sheahan, B., Currie, D., & McKeown, L. (2021). Crossing the border during the pandemic: 2020 in review. Statistics Canada, 23 February. https://www150.statcan.gc.ca/n1/pub/45-28-0001/2021001/article/00007-eng.htm

Arnold, K. R. (2004). *Homelessness, citizenship, and identity: The uncanniness of late modernity*. State University of New York Press.

Atkinson, R. (1998). *The life story interview*. SAGE Publishing.

Awan, K., Sheikh, M., Mithoowani, N., Ahmed, A., & Simard, D. (2007). Maclean's magazine: A case study of media-propagated Islamophobia. Canadian Islamic Congress.

Bailey, M., & Mobley, I. A. (2019). Work in the intersections: A Black feminist disability framework. *Gender & Society*, *33*(1), 19–40. https://doi.org/10.1177/0891243218801523

Bakari, M. A. (2001). *The democratisation process in Zanzibar*. GIGA-Hamburg.

Baker, P., & McEnery, T. (2005). A corpus-based approach to discourses of refugees and asylum seekers in UN and newspaper texts. *Journal of Language and Politics*, *4*(2), 197–226.

Bakke, P., & Kuypers, J. (2016). The Syrian civil war, international outreach, and a clash of worldviews. *The Journal of Kenneth Burke Society*, *11*(2). https://kbjournal.org/bakke-kuypers

Barton, L. (1993). The struggle for citizenship: The case of disabled people. *Disability, Handicap & Society*, *8*(3), 235–248. https://doi.org/10.1080/02674649366780251

Bauman, Z. (1991). *Modernity and ambivalence*. Polity Press.

Beck, E., Charania, M., Abed-Rabo Al-Issa, F., & Wahab, S. (2017). Undoing Islamophobia: Awareness of orientalism in social work. *Journal of Progressive Human Services*, *28*(2), 58–72. https://doi.org/10.1080/10428232.2017.1310542

Beiser, M. (2009). Resettling refugees and safeguarding their mental health: Lessons learned from the Canadian refugee resettlement project. *Transcultural Psychiatry*, *46*(4), 539–583. https://doi.org/10.1177/1363461509351373

Ben-Moshe, L., & Magaña, S. (2014). An introduction to race, gender, and disability: Intersectionality, disability studies, and families of color. *Women, Gender, and Families of Color*, *2*(2), 105–114. https://doi.org/10.5406/womgenfamcol.2.2.0105

Berne, P. (2015). Disability justice – A working draft by Patty Berne. Sins Invalid, 10 June. https://www.sinsinvalid.org/blog/disability-justice-a-working-draft-by-patty-berne

Berne, P., Morales, A. L., Langstaff, D., & Sins Invalid (2018). Ten principles of disability justice. *WSQ: Women's Studies Quarterly, 46*(1), 227–230. https://doi.org/10.1353/wsq.2018.0003

Beydoun, K. (2016). Islamophobia: Toward a legal definition and framework. *Columbia Law Review, 116*(7), 108–125.

Bickenbach, J. E. (2009). Disability, culture and the U.N. convention. *Disability and Rehabilitation, 31*(14), 1111–1124. https://doi.org/10.1080/09638280902773729

Bisset, K. (2016). Trudeau shares refugee family's chocolate business story in UN speech. *The Toronto Star*, 21 September. https://www.thestar.com/news/canada/2016/09/21/trudeau-shares-refugee-familys-chocolate-business-story-in-un-speech.html

Bochner, A., Ellis, C., & Tillmann-Healy, L. (2000). Relationships as stories: Accounts, storied lives, evocative narratives. In K. Dindia & S. Duck (Eds.), *Communication in personal relationships* (pp. 307–324). John Wiley & Sons.

Bose, P. S. (2020). The shifting landscape of international resettlement: Canada, the U.S. and Syrian refugees. *Geopolitics, 27*(2), 375–401. https://doi.org/10.1080/14650045.2020.1781820

Boudjikanian, R. (2021). Federal immigration department employees reporting racist workplace behaviour, says survey. *CBC*, 20 October. https://www.cbc.ca/news/politics/immigration-refugees-citizenship-racism-1.6217886

Bradley, L., & Tawfiq, N. (2006). The physical and psychological effects of torture in Kurds seeking asylum in the United Kingdom. *Torture: Quarterly Journal on Rehabilitation of Torture Victims and Prevention of Torture, 16*(1), 41–47.

Bryant, T., Aquanno, S., & Raphael, D. (2020). Unequal impact of COVID-19: Emergency neoliberalism and welfare policy in Canada. *Critical Studies: An International & Interdisciplinary Journal, 15*(1), 22–39.

Bukar, A. A. (2020). The political economy of hate industry: Islamophobia in the Western public sphere. *Islamophobia Studies Journal, 5*(2), 152–174. https://doi.org/10.13169/islastudj.5.2.0152

Bullock, K., & Zhou, S. (2017). Entertainment or blackface? Decoding Orientalism in a post-9/11 era: Audience views on Aladdin. *Review of Education, Pedagogy, and Cultural Studies, 39*(5), 446–469. https://doi.org/10.1080/10714413.2017.1344512

Burns, N. (2017). The human right to health: Exploring disability, migration and health. *Disability and Society, 32*(10), pp. 1463–1484. https://doi.org/10.1080/09687599.2017.1358604

Burton, P., & Phipps, S. (2009). Economic costs of caring for children with disabilities in Canada. *Canadian Public Policy, 35*(3), 269–290. https://www.jstor.org/stable/40345324

Butler, J. (1993). *Bodies that matter: On the discursive limits of "sex"*. Routledge.
Canadian Council for Refugees (CCR) (2017). 2017 immigration levels comments. http://ccrweb.ca/en/2017-immigration-levels-comments
CCR, Amnesty International Canada, Canadian Association of Refugee Lawyers, & BC Civil Liberties Association (2020). Call for border to be reopened to refugees. 2 April. https://ccrweb.ca/en/media/call-border-be-reopened-refugees-02-04-2020
CBC News (2018). No space in Windsor's temporary shelters for Toronto refugees. CBC, 6 July. https://www.cbc.ca/news/canada/windsor/toronto-refugees-windsor-shelter-1.4737636
CBC Radio (2016). How Syrian refugees arriving in Canada became 'extras' in their own stories. CBC, 19 February. https://www.cbc.ca/radio/the180/how-syrian-refugees-arriving-in-canada-become-extras-in-their-own-stories-1.3452625
Charlton, J. I. (2000). *Nothing about us without us: Disability oppression and empowerment*. University of California Press.
Chen, Y. Y. B., Gruben, V., & Liew, J. C. Y. (2018). 'A legacy of confusion': An exploratory study of service provision under the reinstated interim federal health program. *Refuge: Canada's Journal on Refugees, 34*(2), 94–102. https://doi.org/10.7202/1055580ar
Church, K., Vorstermans, J., & Underwood, K. (2020). Tensions of transinstitutionalization in disabled childhoods: A photo essay. *Canadian Journal of Disability Studies, 9*(3), 120–142. https://doi.org/10.15353/cjds.v9i3.649
Clandinin, D. J. (2006). Narrative inquiry: A methodology for studying lived experience. *Research Studies in Music Education, 27*(1), 44–54. https://doi.org/10.1177/1321103X060270010301
Clandinin, D. J. (2013). *Engaging in narrative inquiry*. Left Coast Press.
Clandinin, D. J., & Connelly, F. M. (2000). *Narrative inquiry: Experience and story in qualitative research*. Jossey-Bass.
Clandinin, D. J., & Rosiek, J. (2007). Mapping a landscape of narrative inquiry: Borderland spaces and tensions. In D. J. Clandinin (Ed.), *Handbook of narrative inquiry: Mapping a methodology* (pp. 35–75). SAGE Publishing.
Clandinin, D. J., Murphy, M. S., & Huber, J. (2011). *Places of curriculum making: Narrative inquiries into children's lives in motion*. Emerald Group Publishing Limited.
Comeau, É., Kelly, S., Hamdani, Y., & Ross, T. (2024). Disabled people's accessible taxi experiences in Toronto, Canada. *Travel Behaviour and Society, 34*, 100704. https://doi.org/10.1016/j.tbs.2023.100704

Connelly, F. M., & Clandinin, D. J. (2006). Narrative inquiry. In J. Green, G. Camilli, & P. Elmore (Eds.), *Handbook of complementary methods in education research* (Rev. ed., pp. 375–385). Routledge.

Council of Canadians with Disabilities (CCD). (2012). Immigration and people with disabilities. http://www.ccdonline.ca/en/socialpolicy/immigration

Crenshaw, K. (1991). Mapping the margins: Intersectionality, identity politics, and violence against women of color. In K. Crenshaw, N. Gotanda, G. Peller, & K. Thomas (Eds.), *Critical race theory: The key writings that formed the movement* (pp. 357–383). The New Press.

Crenshaw, K. W. (1995). Mapping the margins: The intersection of race and gender. In K. W. Crenshaw, N. Gotanda, G. Peller, & K. Thomas (Eds.), *Critical race theory* (pp. 357–383). The New Press.

Crenshaw, K. (1998). Demarginalizing the intersection of race and sex: A Black feminist critique of antidiscrimination doctrine, feminist theory, and antiracist politics. In A. Phillips (Ed.), *Feminism and politics* (pp. 314–343). Oxford University Press.

Crenshaw, K. (2016). The urgency of intersectionality [Video]. YouTube, 7 December. https://www.youtube.com/watch?v=akOe5-UsQ2oandlist=PLOGi5-fAu8bHEkVWA2JbDFnpARSUqX0Rw

Crock, M., Ernst, C., & McCallum, R. (2012). Where disability and displacement intersect: Asylum seekers and refugees with disabilities. *International Journal of Refugee Law, 24*(4), 735–764.

Crock, M., Smith-Khan, L., McCallum, R. C., & Saul, B. (2017). *The legal protection of refugees with disabilities: Forgotten and invisible?* Edward Elgar Publishing.

Danso, R. (2002). From 'there' to 'here': An investigation of the initial settlement experiences of Ethiopian and Somali refugees in Toronto. *GeoJournal, 56*(1), 3–14.

Davis, L. (1999). Riding with the man on the escalator: Citizenship and disability. In L. A. Basser Marks, & M. Jones (Eds.), *Disability, divers-ability and legal change* (pp. 65–73). Brill.

Dawson, A. C. (2019). Stasis in flight: Reframing disability and dependence in the refugee. *Disability Studies Quarterly, 39*(1). https://doi.org/10.18061/dsq.v39i1

Degener, T. (2016). Disability in a human rights context. *Laws, 5*(3), 35. https://doi.org/10.3390/laws5030035

DeJonckheere, M., & Vaughn, L. M. (2019). Semistructured interviewing in primary care research: A balance of relationship and rigour. *Family Medicine and Community Health, 7*(2), e000057. https://doi.org/10.1136/fmch-2018-000057

Dhamoon, R. K. (2011). Considerations on mainstreaming intersectionality. *Political Research Quarterly, 64*(1), 230–243. https://doi.org/10.1177/1065912910379227

Donato, K.M., & Ferris, E. (2020). Refugee integration in Canada, Europe, and the United States: Perspectives from research. *The Annals of the American Academy of Political and Social Science, 690*(1), 7–35. https://doi.org/10.1177/0002716220943169

Dossa, P. (2008). Creating politicized spaces: Afghan immigrant women's stories of migration and displacement. *Affilia, 23*(1), 10–21. https://doi.org/10.1177/0886109907310462

Dossa, P. (2009). *Racialized bodies, disabling worlds: Storied lives of immigrant Muslim women.* University of Toronto Press.

Dossa, P. (2013). Structural violence in Afghanistan: Gendered memory, narratives, and food. *Medical Anthropology, 32*(5), 433–447. https://doi.org/10.1080/01459740.2012.721826

Dossa, P. (2018). From displaced care to social care: Narrative interventions of Canadian Muslims. *American Anthropologist, 120*(3), 558–560. https://doi.org/10.1111/aman.13095

Earle, A., & Heymann, J. (2012). The cost of caregiving: Wage loss among caregivers of elderly and disabled adults and children with special needs. *Community, Work & Family, 15*(3), 357-375.

Edmonds, J., & Flahault, A. (2021). Refugees in Canada during the first wave of the COVID-19 pandemic. *International Journal of Environmental Research and Public Health, 18*(3), 947. https://doi.org/10.3390/ijerph18030947

Elder, B. C. (2015). Stories from the margins: Refugees with disabilities rebuilding lives. *Societies without Borders, 10*(1), 1–27.

Elkassem, S., Csiernik, R., Mantulak, A., Kayssi, G., Hussain, Y., Lambert, K., Bailey, P., & Choudhary, A. (2018). Growing up Muslim: The impact of Islamophobia on children in a Canadian community. *Journal of Muslim Mental Health, 12*(1), 3–18. https://doi.org/10.3998/jmmh.10381607.0012.101

El-Lahib, Y., & Wehbi, S. (2012). Immigration and disability: Ableism in the policies of the Canadian state. *International Social Work, 55*(1), 95–108.

Erevelles, N. (2002). (Im)Material citizens: Cognitive disability, race, and the politics of citizenship. In M. Wappett & K. Arndt (Eds.), *Foundations of disability studies* (pp. 145–176). Palgrave Macmillan.

Erevelles, N. (2011). *Disability and difference in global contexts: Enabling a transformative body politic.* Palgrave Macmillan.

Erevelles, N. (2014). Thinking with disability studies. *Disability Studies Quarterly, 34*(2). https://doi.org/10.18061/dsq.v34i2.4248

Essed, P. (1991). *Understanding everyday racism: An interdisciplinary theory*. SAGE Publishing.
Farmer, P. (2003). *Pathologies of power: Structural violence and the assault on human rights*. University of California Press.
Farmer, P. (2005). *Pathologies of power: Health, human rights, and the new war on the poor*. University of California Press.
Fernando, S., & Rinaldi, J. (2017). Seeking equity: Disrupting a history of exclusionary immigration frameworks. *Canadian Ethnic Studies, 49*(3), 7–26.
Fouad, F. M., McCall, S. J., Ayoub, H., Abu-Raddad, L. J., & Mumtaz, G. R. (2021). Vulnerability of Syrian refugees in Lebanon to COVID-19: Quantitative insights. *Conflict and Health, 15,* 13. https://doi.org/10.1186/s13031-021-00349-6
Frank, A. W. (2000). The standpoint of storyteller. *Qualitative Health Research, 10*(3), 354–365.
Frank, G. (2000). *Venus on wheels: Two decades of dialogue on disability, biography and being female in America*. University of California Press.
Gangamma, R., & Shipman, D. (2018). Transnational intersectionality in family therapy with resettled refugees. *Journal of Family Therapy, 44*(2), 206–219.
Garland-Thomson, R. (1997). *Extraordinary bodies: Figuring physical disability in American culture and literature*. Columbia University Press.
Globe and Mail (2015). Canadian military flight brings Canada's first planeload of Syrian refugees to Toronto. 11 December https://www.theglobeandmail.com/news/national/canadian-military-flight-brings-canadas-first-planeload-of-syrian-refugees-to-toronto/article27710746/
Goodley, D., & Lawthom, R. (2019). Critical disability studies, Brexit and Trump: A time of neoliberal–ableism. *Rethinking History, 23*(2), 233–251. https://doi.org/10.1080/13642529.2019.1607476
Gorman, R. J. K. (2005). Class consciousness, disability, and social exclusion: A relational/reflexive analysis of disability culture [Doctoral dissertation, University of Toronto].
Gorman, R. (2007). The feminist standpoint and the trouble with 'informal learning': A way forward for Marxist-Feminist educational research. In A. Green, G. Rikowski, & H. Raduntz (Eds.), *Renewing dialogues in Marxism and education* (pp. 183–199). Palgrave Macmillan. https://doi.org/10.1057/9780230609679_10
Gorman, R. (2016). Disablement in and for itself: Towards a 'global' idea of disability. *Somatechnics, 6*(2), 249–261. https://doi.org/10.3366/soma.2016.0194

Gorman, R. (2018). Dialectics of race and disability: On the unintelligibility of revolutionary desire. *a.b: Auto/Biography Studies, 33*(2), 453–458.

Government of Canada (2016). Canada's private sponsorship of refugees program. https://www.canada.ca/en/immigration-refugees-citizenship/news/2016/09/canada-private-sponsorship-refugees-program.html

Government of Canada (2018). Trauma and violence-informed approaches to policy and practice. https://www.canada.ca/en/public-health/services/publications/health-risks-safety/trauma-violence-informed-approaches-policy-practice.html

Government of Canada (2020a). By the numbers – 40 years of Canada's Private Sponsorship of Refugees Program. https://www.canada.ca/en/immigration-refugees-citizenship/news/2019/04/by-the-numbers--40-years-of-canadas-private-sponsorship-of-refugees-program.html

Government of Canada (2020b). Promoting rights of persons with disabilities. https://www.international.gc.ca/world-monde/issues_development-enjeux_developpement/human_rights-droits_homme/rights_disabilities-droits_handicapees.aspx?lang=eng

Government of Canada (2022a). Disability in Canada: A 2006 profile. https://www.canada.ca/en/employment-social-development/programs/disability/arc/disability-2006.html#s3

Government of Canada (2022b). Excessive demand on health services and social services. https://www.canada.ca/en/immigration-refugees-citizenship/corporate/publications-manuals/operational-bulletins-manuals/standard-requirements/medical-requirements/refusals-inadmissibility/excessive-demand-on-health-social-services.html

Government of Canada (2022c). Statement from the Chief Public Health Officer of Canada on January 21, 2022. https://www.canada.ca/en/public-health/news/2022/01/statement-from-the-chief-public-health-officer-of-canada-on-january-21-2022.html

Government of Canada (2024). #WelcomeRefugees: Key figures. https://www.canada.ca/en/immigration-refugees-citizenship/services/refugees/about-refugee-system/welcome-syrian-refugees/key-figures.html

Gowayed, H. (2020). Resettled and unsettled: Syrian refugees and the intersection of race and legal status in the United States. *Ethnic and Racial Studies, 43*(2), 275–293. https://doi.org/10.1080/01419870.2019.1583350

Gravelle, T. (2018). Friends, neighbours, townspeople and parties: Explaining Canadian attitudes toward Muslims. *Canadian Journal of Political Science, 51*(3), 643–664.

Grech, S., & Soldatic, K. (2015). Disability and colonialism: (Dis)encounters and anxious intersectionalities. *Social Identities, 21*(1), 1–5. https://doi.org/10.1080/13504630.2014.995394

Hahn, H. (1985). Toward a politics of disability: Definitions, disciplines, and policies. *The Social Science Journal, 22*(4), 87–105.

Hakeem, O., & Jabri, S. (2015). Adverse birth outcomes in women exposed to Syrian chemical attack. *The Lancet Global Health, 3*(4), e196. https://doi.org/10.1016/S2214-109X(15)70077-X

Hankivsky, O. (Ed.) (2012). *An intersectionality-based policy analysis framework*. Institute for Intersectionality Research & Policy, Simon Fraser University.

Harell, A. (2017). Intersectionality and gendered political behaviour in a multicultural Canada. *Canadian Journal of Political Science/Revue canadienne de science politique, 50*(2), 495–514. https://doi.org/10.1017/S000842391700021X

Hasford, J. (2016). Dominant cultural narratives, racism, and resistance in the workplace: A study of the experiences of young black Canadians. *American Journal of Community Psychology, 57*(1–2), 158–170.

Haugen, S. (2019). 'We feel like we're home': The resettlement and integration of Syrian refugees in smaller and rural Canadian communities. *Refuge: Canada's Journal on Refugees, 35*(2), 53–63. https://doi.org/10.7202/1064819ar

Hays, D. G., & Singh, A. A. (2012). *Qualitative inquiry in clinical and educational settings*. Guilford Press.

Heibert, D. (2016). What's so special about Canada? Understanding the resilience of immigration and multiculturalism. Washington, DC: Migration Policy Institute. https://nsiip.ca/wp-content/uploads/Hiebert_whats-so-special-about-Canada.pdf

Hill Collins, P., & Bilge, S. (2016). *Intersectionality*. Polity Press.

Houle, R. (2019). Results from the 2016 census: Syrian refugees who resettled in Canada in 2015 and 2016. Insights on Canadian Society, Statistics Canada. https://www150.statcan.gc.ca/n1/en/pub/75-006-x/2019001/article/00001-eng.pdf?st=ygB1Mjs8

Hughes, B. (2014). Disabled people as counterfeit citizens: The politics of resentment past and present. *Disability & Society, 30*(7), 991–1004.

Hughes, S. E. (2019). #WelcomeToCanada: Performing asylum, defending nation. *Canadian Theatre Review, 177*, 14–19. https://doi.org/10.3138/ctr.177.003

Humanity and Inclusion (2015). 1/5 Syrian refugees has disability. https://hi-canada.org/en/news/1-5-syrian-refugees-has-disability-

Hyndman, J. (2011). A refugee camp conundrum: Geopolitics, liberal democracy, and protracted refugee situation. *Refuge, 28*(2), 7–15.

Hyndman, J., Payne, W., & Jimenez, S. (2017). Private refugee sponsorship in Canada. *Forced Migration Review, 54*, 56–59.

Hynie, M. (2018). Canada's Syrian refugee program, intergroup relationships and identities. *Canadian Ethnic Studies, 50*(2), 1–12. https://doi.org/10.1353/ces.2018.0012

Ingstad, B., & Whyte, R. (Eds.) (2007). *Disability in local and global worlds*. University of California.

Iyase, B. N., & Folarin, S. F. (2018). A critique of veto power system in the United Nations Security Council. *ACTA UNIVERSITATIS DANUBIUS: International Relations, 11*(2), 104-122.

Immigration, Refugees and Citizenship Canada (IRCC). (2022). Questions and answers by topic: Refugee sponsorship. Government of Canada. Retrieved November 25, 2023, from https://ircc.canada.ca/english/helpcentre/questions-answers-by-topic.asp?top=11

Issari, P., Christopoulou, A., & Galika, A. (2021). Life stories of Syrian refugees: A qualitative study. *Psychology, 12*(10), 1542–1560. https://doi.org/10.4236/psych.2021.1210097.

Jaeger, P. T., & Bowman, C. A. (2005). *Understanding disability: Inclusion, access, diversity, and civil rights*. Praeger.

Jampel, C. (2018). Intersections of disability justice, racial justice and environmental justice. *Environmental Sociology, 4*(1), 122–135. https://doi.org/10.1080/23251042.2018.1424497

Janoski, T., & Gran, B. (2002). Political citizenship: Foundations of rights. In E. Isin & B. Turner (Eds.), *Handbook of citizenship studies*. SAGE Publishing.

Kaida, L., Hou, F., & Stick, M. (2020). The long-term economic integration of resettled refugees in Canada: A comparison of privately sponsored refugees and government-assisted refugees. *Journal of Ethnic and Migration Studies, 46*(9), 1687–1708. https://doi.org/10.1080/1369183X.2019.1623017

Kamran, N. (2023). *Private refugee sponsorship in Canada: Sharing the lessons of a good practice*. KNOMAD, World Bank Group.

Karsay, D., & Lewis, O. (2012). Disability, torture and ill-treatment: Taking stock and ending abuses. *The International Journal of Human Rights, 16*(6), 816–830. https://doi.org/10.1080/13642987.2012.718506

Kayess, R., & French, P. (2008). Out of darkness into light? Introducing the Convention on the Rights of Persons with Disabilities. *Human Rights Law Review, 8*(1), 1–34.

Kazemi, S. (2018). Toward a conceptualization of transnational disability theory and praxis: Entry point, Iraqi chemical attack on Iran [Doctoral dissertation, University of Toronto].

Kazemi, S. (2019). Disabling power of class and ideology: Analyzing war injury through the transnational disability theory and praxis. *Disability Studies Quarterly, 39*(3). https://doi.org/10.18061/dsq.v39i3.6496

Kazimi, A. (2012). *The undesirables: White Canada and the Komagata Maru: An illustrated history.* Douglas & McIntyre.

Kerwin, D. (2016). How robust refugee protection policies can strengthen human and national security. *Journal on Migration and Human Security, 4*(3), 83–140. https://doi.org/10.1177/233150241600400304

Kett, M., & Van Ommeren, M. (2009). Disability, conflict, and emergencies. *The Lancet, 374*(9704), 1801–1803.

Khafaei, M., Panahi, Y., Abolghasemi, H., Miri, A., Karimi, F., & Farnoosh, G. (2024). Injuries Caused by White Phosphorus Bombing as a Crisis in Gaza Strip. *Trauma Monthly, 29*(1), 1052-1057. doi: 10.30491/tm.2024.452290.1719

Kluge, H. H. P., Jakab, Z., Bartovic, J., D'Anna, V., & Severoni, S. (2020). Refugee and migrant health in the COVID-19 response. *The Lancet, 395*(10232), 1237–1239. https://doi.org/10.1016/S0140-6736(20)30791-1

Kofman, E. (Ed.) (2000). *Gender and international migration in Europe: Employment, welfare, and politics.* Routledge.

Kruglanski, A., Webber, D., Molinario, E., & Jaśko, K. (2019). Are Syrian refugees a danger to the West? The Conversation, 19 July. https://theconversation.com/are-syrian-refugees-a-danger-to-the-west-113803

Labman, S. (2016). Private sponsorship: Complementary or conflicting interests? *Refuge: Canada's Journal on Refugees, 32*(2), 67–80. https://doi.org/10.25071/1920-7336.40266

Lanphier, M. (2003). Sponsorship: Organizational, sponsor, and refugee perspectives. *Journal of International Migration and Integration / Revue de l'integration et de La Migration Internationale, 4*(2), 237–256. https://doi.org/10.1007/s12134-003-1035-x

Lawlor, C., & Mattingly, M. (2000). Learning from stories: Narrative interviewing in cross-cultural research. *Scandinavian Journal of Occupational Therapy, 7*(1), 4–14. https://doi.org/10.1080/110381200443571

Liptak, A., & Shear, M. D. (June 26, 2018). Trump's travel ban is upheld by Supreme Court. *The New York Times.* https://www.nytimes.com/2018/06/26/us/politics/supreme-court-trump-travel-ban.html

Levy, S. (2019, November 29). Refugees will cost Toronto taxpayers $75M this year. *Toronto Sun.* https://torontosun.com/news/local-news/levyrefugees-will-cost-toronto-taxpayers-75m-this-year

Maclean's. (2020, April 13), Doug Ford's April 13 Ontario coronavirus update: Full replay. [Video]. Maclean's. https://www.macleans.ca/news/canada/doug-fords-april-13-ontario coronavirus-update-live-video/

March of Dimes Canada. (2024). *HVMP - What We Fund.* https://www.marchofdimes.ca/en-ca/programs/am/hvmp/Pages/HVMP-Funding.aspx

Massfeller, H., & Hamm, L. D. (2019). "I'm thinking I want to live a better life": Syrian refugee student adjustment in New Brunswick. *Journal of Contemporary Issues in Education, 14*(1). https://doi.org/10.20355/jcie29354

McMahon, M. (2007). Life story counselling: Producing new identities in career counselling. In J. G. Maree (Ed.), *Shaping the story: A guide to facilitating narrative career counselling* (pp. 62–71). Van Schaik Publishers.

Meekosha, H. (2008). Contextualizing disability: Developing southern theory. Keynote address presented at the Fourth Disability Studies Association Conference, University of Lancaster, Lancaster, UK. 2–4 September.

Meekosha, H., & Soldatic, K. (2011). Social model of disability. In R. K. McRuer & A. M. K. L. O. (Eds.), *Disability studies: A reader* (pp. 56–68). Routledge.

Mirza, M. (2011). Disability and humanitarianism in refugee camps: The case for a travelling supranational disability praxis. *Third World Quarterly, 32*(8), 1527–1536. https://doi.org/10.1080/01436597.2011.604524

Mollica, R. F. (2001). The trauma story: A phenomenological approach to the traumatic life experiences of refugee survivors. *Psychiatry, 64*(1), 60–72. https://doi.org/10.1521/psyc.64.1.60.18242

Moore, A. S. (2022). *Violent exceptions: Children's human rights and humanitarian rhetorics* by Wendy S. Hesford (review). *Human Rights Quarterly 44*(3), 640–644. https://dx.doi.org/10.1353/hrq.2022.0030.

Morris, J. (2001). Impairment and disability: Constructing an ethics of care that promotes human rights. *Hypatia, A Journal of Feminist Philosophy, 16*(4), 1–16.

Morris, J. (2005). Citizenship and disabled people: A scoping paper prepared for the Disability Rights Commission.

Mothoagae, O. (2018). The false archive: A space of re-collection, re-writing and re-imaging [Doctoral dissertation, University of Johannesburg].

Mullings, D. V., Morgan, A., & Quelleng, H. K. (2016). Canada the great white north where anti-black racism thrives: Kicking down the doors and exposing the realities. *Phylon, 53*(1), 20–41. https://www.jstor.org/stable/phylon1960.53.1.20

Nagi, Y., Sender, H., Orcutt, M., Fouad, F., Burgess, R. A., & Devakumar, D. (2021). Resilience as a communal concept: Understanding adolescent resilience in the context of the Syrian refugee crisis in Bar Elias, Lebanon. *Journal of Migration and Health, 3*, 100046. https://doi.org/10.1016/j.jmh.2021.100046

National Assembly of Québec (2019). Bill 21: An act respective the laicity of the state. https://ccla.org/wp-content/uploads/2021/09/2019-06-16-Bill-21-Passes-and-Becomes-Law.pdf

National Council of Canadian Muslims (NCCM) (2021). NCCM recommendations: National Summit on Islamophobia. https://www.nccm.ca/wp-content/uploads/2021/06/Policy-Recommendations_NCCM.pdf

Neuman, K. (2016). *Survey of Muslims in Canada 2016: Final Report*. Toronto: Environics Institute. https://www.environicsinstitute.org/docs/default-source/project-documents/survey-of-muslims-in-canada-2016/final-report.pdf

Newborn Screening Ontario (2021). Newborn Screening Manual. A guide for newborn care providers. https://www.newborn-screening.on.ca/en/publications/newborn-screening-manual

Norris, T. (2021). Memorialization, decolonization, and schools: Memorializing forced forgetting. *A Journal of Educational Research and Practice, 31*(1), 1–6. https://doi.org/10.26522/brocked.v31i1.950

Oliver, M. (1992). Education for citizenship: Issues for further education. The Walter Lessing Memorial Lecture. https://disability-studies.leeds.ac.uk/wp-content/uploads/sites/40/library/Oliver-walter-lessing.pdf

Oliver, M. (2004). The social model in action: If I had a hammer. In C. Barnes and G. Mercer (Eds.), *Implementing the social model of disability: Theory and research* (pp. 18–31). The Disability Press.

Oliver, M., & Barnes, C. (2012). *The new politics of disablement*. Palgrave Macmillan.

Olsen, C., El-Bialy, R., Mckelvie, M., Rauman, P., & Brunger, F. (2016). 'Other' troubles: Deconstructing perceptions and changing responses to refugees in Canada. *Journal of Immigrant and Minority Health*, *18*(1), 58–66. https://doi.org/10.1007/s10903-014-9983-0

Olsen, R., & Clarke, H. (2003). *Parenting and disability: Disabled parents' experiences of raising children*. Policy Press.

Ontario Human Rights Commission (2001). An intersectional approach to discrimination: Addressing multiple grounds in human rights claims. https://www3.ohrc.on.ca/sites/default/files/attachments/An_intersectional_approach_to_discrimination%3A_Addressing_multiple_grounds_in_human_rights_claims.pdf

Ontario Human Rights Commission (2016). Policy on ableism and discrimination based on disability. https://www.ohrc.on.ca/sites/default/files/Policy%20on%20ableism%20and%20discrimination%20based%20on%20disability_accessible_2016.pdf

Ontario Ministry of Education (2018). Identifying students with special education needs http://www.edu.gov.on.ca/eng/general/elemsec/speced/individu.html

Oudshoorn, A., Benbow, S., & Meyer, M. (2020). Resettlement of Syrian refugees in Canada. *Journal of International Migration and Integration*, *21*(3), 893–908. https://doi.org/10.1007/s12134-019-00695-8

Parchomiuk, M. (2014). Social context of disabled parenting. *Sexuality and Disability*, *32*(2), 231–242. https://doi.org/10.1007/s111

Pisani, M. (2012). Addressing the 'citizenship assumption' in critical pedagogy: exploring the case of rejected female sub-Saharan African asylum seekers in Malta. *Power and Education*, *4*(2), 185–195.

Pisani, M., & Grech, S. (2015). Disability and forced migration: critical intersectionalities. *Disability and the Global South*, *2*(1), 421–441.

Pope, C., & Mays, N. (Eds.) (2006). *Qualitative research in health care*. Blackwell Publishing Ltd. https://doi.org/10.1002/9780470750841

Pottie, K., Greenaway, C., Hassan, G., Hui, C., & Kirmayer, L. J. (2016). Caring for a newly arrived Syrian refugee family. *Canadian Medical Association Journal*, *188*(3), 207–211. https://doi.org/10.1503/cmaj.151422

Press Progress (2021). Doug Ford's 2021 Budget Confirms Over $1 Billion in Cuts to Education, Ontario School Board Says. 24 March. https://pressprogress.ca/doug-fords-2021-budget-confirms-over-1-billion-in-cuts-to-education-ontario-school-boards-say

Prince, M. J. (2004). Disability, disability studies and citizenship: Moving up or off the sociological agenda? *The Canadian Journal of Sociology*, *29*(3), 459–467.

Prince, M. J. (2009). *Absent citizens: Disability politics and policy in Canada*. University of Toronto Press.

Puar, J. (2017). *The right to maim: Debility, capacity, disability*. Duke University Press.

Public Health Ontario (2021). Enhanced epidemiological summary. https://www.publichealthontario.ca/-/media/documents/ncov/epi/covid-19-regional-epi-summary-report.pdf?sc_lang=en.

Rahman, M. (2017). *Islamophobia, the impossible Muslim, and the reflexive potential of intersectionality*. Routledge.

Rajaram, P. K., & Grundy-Warr, C. (Eds.) (2007). *Borderscapes: Hidden geographies and politics at territory's edge*. University of Minnesota Press.

Ramirez, E. G. (2021). Diversity, equity, and inclusion: Is it just another catchphrase? *Advanced Emergency Nursing Journal, 43*(2), 87–88. https://doi.org/10.1097/TME.0000000000000353

Rawls, J. (1998). Justice as fairness in the liberal polity. In G. Shafir (Ed.), *The citizenship debates: A reader* (pp. 53–72). University of Minnesota Press.

Razack, S. H. (1998). *Looking white people in the eye: Gender, race, and culture in courtrooms and classrooms*. University of Toronto Press.

Razack, S. H (2013). Timely deaths: Medicalizing the deaths of Aboriginal people in police custody. *Law, Culture, and the Humanities, 9*(2), 352–374. https://doi.org/10.1177/1743872111407022

Refugee Sponsorship Training Program (RSTP). (2018). *Sponsorship cost table*. Infosheets. Retrieved March 5, 2023, from https://www.rstp.ca/en/infosheet/sponsorship-cost-table-2/

Reilly, R. (2010). Disabilities among refugees and conflict-affected populations. *Forced Review, 35*, 8–10.

Rettberg, J. W., & Gajjala, R. (2015). Terrorists or cowards: Negative portrayals of male Syrian refugees in social media. *Feminist Media Studies, 16*(1), 178–181. https://doi.org/10.1080/14680777.2016.1120493

Rioux, M., & Carbert, A. (2003). Human rights and disability: The international context. *Journal on Developmental Disabilities, 10*(2), 1–13.

Rioux, M. H., & Valentine, F. (2006). Does theory matter? Exploring the nexus between disability, human rights and public policy. In R. F. Devlin & D. Pothier (Eds.), *Critical disability theory: Essays in philosophy, politics, policy, and law* (pp. 47–69). UBC Press.

Rioux, M. H., Basser Marks, L. A., & Jones, M. (2011). *Critical perspectives on human rights and disability law*. Brill | Nijhoff. https://doi.org/10.1163/ej.9789004189508.i-552.

Rioux, M.H., Prince, M.J. (2002). The Canadian political landscape of disability: Policy perspectives, social status, interest groups, and the rights movement. In A. Putee (Ed.), *Federalism, democracy and disability policy in Canada* (pp. 11–29). McGill-Queen's University Press.

Rolston, Y. (2014). Are you disabled? Social and cultural factors in understanding disability in Trinidad and Tobago [Doctoral dissertation, London Metropolitan University]. https://core.ac.uk/download/96599422.pdf

Rose, A. C. (2020). Blackness and disability and how disability is too often forgotten [Student research paper, Gettysburg College]. https://cupola.gettysburg.edu/student_scholarship/863

Rukavina, S. (2022). New research shows Bill 21 having 'devastating' impact on religious minorities in Quebec: Survey shows most Quebec Muslims feel less accepted, less safe and less hopeful under new law. CBC News, 4 August. https://www.cbc.ca/news/canada/montreal/bill-21-impact-religious-minorities-1.6540400

Russell, M. (2002). What disability civil rights cannot do: Employment and political economy. *Disability & Society*, *17*(2), 117–135. https://doi.org/10.1080/09687590120122288

Ryu, M., & Tuvilla, M. R. S. (2018). Resettled refugee youths' stories of migration, schooling, and future: Challenging dominant narratives about refugees. *The Urban Review*, *50*(4), 539–558. https://doi.org/10.1007/s11256-018-0455-z

Sakellariou, D., & Pollard, N. (2016). *Occupational therapies without borders: Integrating justice with practice* (2nd ed.). Elsevier.

Said, W. E. (1978). *Orientalism*. Random House

Said, W. E. (2000). *Reflections on Exile and Other Essays*. Harvard University Press.

Saleh, M. (2017). *Stories we live by, with, in: A narrative inquiry into the experiences of Canadian Muslim girls and their mothers* [doctoral thesis]. University of Alberta.

Saleh, M. (2019). *Stories we live and grow by: (Re)Telling our experiences as Muslim mothers and daughters*. Demeter Press.

Schack, L., & Witcher, A. (2021). Hostile hospitality and the criminalization of civil society actors aiding border crossers in Greece. *EPD: Society and Space*, *39*(3), 477–495. https://doi.org/10.1177/0263775820958709

Schur, L., Kruse, D., & Blanck, P. D. (2013). *People with disabilities: Sidelined or mainstreamed?* Cambridge University Press.

Scribner, T. (2017). You are not welcome here anymore: Restoring support for refugee resettlement in the age of Trump. *Journal on Migration and Human Security*, *5*(2), 263–284. https://doi.org/10.1177/233150241700500203

Scott, C., & Safdar, S. (2017). Threat and prejudice against Syrian refugees in Canada: Assessing the moderating effects of multiculturalism, interculturalism, and assimilation. *International Journal of Intercultural Relations, 60*, 28-39.

Sen, A. (2009). *The Idea of Justice*. Harvard University Press.

Shakespeare, T. (2010). The social model of disability. In L. J. Davis (Ed.), *The Disability Studies Reader* (pp. 266–273). Routledge.

Soldatic, K. (2013). The transnational sphere of justice: Disability praxis and the politics of impairment. *Disability and Society, 28*(6), 744–755.

Soldatic, K., & Biyanwila, J. (2006). *Disability and Development: A Critical Southern Standpoint on Able-Bodied Masculinity*. TASA Conference.

Soldatic, K., & Fiske, L. (2009). Bodies 'locked up": Intersections of disability and race in Australian immigration. *Disability and Society, 24*(3), 289–301.

Smart, J. F. (2005). Challenges to the biomedical model of disability: Changes to the practice of rehabilitation counseling. *Directions in Rehabilitation Counseling, 16*(4), 33–43.

Smith, S. J. (2019). Challenging Islamophobia in Canada: Non-Muslim social workers as allies with the Muslim community. *Journal of Social Work Education, 55*(1), 27–46. https://doi.org/10.1080/15426432.2019.1651240

Starr, P. (1982). *The Social Transformation of American Medicine*. Basic Books.

Stienstra, D. (2018). Canadian disability policies in a world of inequalities. *Societies, 8*(2), 36. https://doi.org/10.3390/soc8020036

Stolee, G., & Caton, S. (2018). Twitter, Trump, and the base: A shift to a new form of presidential talk? *Signs and Society, 6*(1), 147–165.

Taleb, Z. B., Bahelah, R., Fouad, F. M., Coutts, A., Wilcox, M., & Maziak, W. (2015). Syria: Health in a country undergoing tragic transition. *International Journal of Public Health, 60*(S1), 63–72. https://doi.org/10.1007/s00038-014-0586-2

Thobani, S. (2007). *Exalted subjects: Studies in the making of race and nation in Canada*. University of Toronto Press.

Taccone, A. (2021, June 9). What we know about the man accused in the London, Ont. Attack. *CTV News*. https://london.ctvnews.ca/what we-know-about-the-man-accused-in-the-london-ont-attack-1.5461538

Tanfani, J. (2016, October 19). Donald Trump Warns That Syrian Refugees Represent 'a Great Trojan Horse' to the U.S. *Los Angeles Times*. https://www.latimes.com/politics/la-na-pol-syrian-refugees-debate 20161019-snap-story.html

Tyyska, V., Blower, J., Deboer, S., Kawai, S., & Walcott, A. (2018). Canadian media coverage of the Syrian refugee crisis: Representation, response, and resettlement. *Geopolitics, History, and International Relations*, *10*(1), 148–166. https://www.jstor.org/stable/26803985

United Nations (2006). Convention on the rights of persons with disabilities (Art. 11). https://www.un.org/disabilities/documents/convention/convoptprot-e.pdf

United Nations (2023). UN calls for immediate ceasefire in Gaza amid humanitarian crisis. 10 November. https://news.un.org/en/story/2023/11/1143672

United Nations (2024). Gaza: Number of children killed higher than from four years of world conflict. 13 March. https://news.un.org/en/story/2024/03/1147512

United Nations Children's Fund (UNICEF) (2020). The secretary-general appeal for global cease-fire: The fury of the virus illustrates the folly of war. 23 March. https://www.unicef.org/yemen/press-releases/secretary-general-appeal-global-cease-fire

United Nations Refugee Agency (UNHCR) (2018). Canada's resettlement levels and global resettlement needs 2018. https://www.unhcr.ca/wp-content/uploads/2017/11/Canada-Refugee-Resettlement-numbers-2018-2020.6.pdf.

UNHCR (2020). Syria regional refugee response. https://data2.unhcr.org/en/situations/syria#_ga=2.115689286.1120363714.1587065689-968033415.1586509661.

UNHCR (2021b). UNHCR – Syria emergency. https://www.unhcr.org/syria emergency.html.

UNHCR (2022). What is the private sponsorship of refugees? https://www.unhcr.ca/in-canada/other-immigration-pathways-refugees/private-sponsorship-refugees/

UNHCR (2024a). Syria refugee crisis explained. https://www.unrefugees.org/news/syria-refugee-crisis-explained/#When%20did%20the%20Syrian%20refugee%20crisis%20begin?

UNHCR (2024b). The 1951 Refugee Convention. https://www.unhcr.org/about-unhcr/overview/1951-refugee-convention

Van Houten, D., & Jacobs, G. (2005). The empowerment of marginals: Strategic paradoxes. *Disability & Society*, *20*(6), 641–654. https://doi.org/10.1080/09687590500249066

Vanhala, L. (2010). *Making rights a reality? Disability rights activists and legal mobilization*. Cambridge University Press.

Veracini, L. (2015). *The settler colonial present*. Palgrave Macmillan.

Walliman, N. (2006). *Sage course companions: Social research methods*. SAGE Publications Ltd.

Webster, L., & Mertova, P. (2007). *Using narrative inquiry as a research method*. Routledge.

Whalley Hammell, K. R. (2015). Client-centred occupational therapy: The importance of critical perspectives. *Scandinavian Journal of Occupational Therapy, 22*(4), 237–243. https://doi.org/10.3109/11038128.2015.1004103

White, M., & Epston, D. (1990). *Narrative means to therapeutic ends*. W. W. Norton.

White House Office Press Secretary (2017). Executive Order: Protecting the nation from foreign terrorist entry into the United States. 27 January. http://www.gdr-elsj.eu/wp-content/uploads/2017/02/EXECUTIVE-ORDER-PROTECTING-THE-NATION-...NTO-THE-UNITED-STATES-whitehouse.gov_.pdf

Wilkins-Laflamme, S. (2018). Islamophobia in Canada: Measuring the realities of negative attitudes toward Muslims and religious discrimination. *Canadian Review of Sociology/Revue Canadienne de Sociologie, 55*(1), 86–110. https://doi.org/10.1111/cars.12180

Wilkinson, L., & Garcea, J. (2017). *The economic integration of refugees in Canada: A mixed record*. Transatlantic Council on Migration, Migration Policy Institute. https://www.migrationpolicy.org/sites/default/files/publications/TCM-Asylum_Canada-FINAL.pdf

Williams, R. C. (2023). From ACEs to early relational health: Implications for clinical practice. *Paediatrics & Child Health, 28*(6), 377–384. https://doi.org/10.1016/j.pedhc.2023.04.002

Willingham, A. J. (2021). Here's what happened – and how – on one of America's darkest days. CNN, 7 January. https://www.cnn.com/2021/01/07/us/five-things-january-7-trnd/index.html

Women's Refugee Commission (2013). *Disability inclusion in the Syrian refugee response in Lebanon*. New York: Women's Refugee Commission. https://reliefweb.int/sites/reliefweb.int/files/resources/Disability_Inclusion_in_the_Syrian_Refugee_Response_in_Lebanon.pdf

World Health Organization (WHO) (2015). *WHO global disability action plan. Better health for all people with disability*. Geneva: WHO. https://www.who.int/publications/i/item/who-global-disability-action-plan-2014-2021

WHO (2020). A virus that respects no borders: Protecting refugees and migrants during COVID-19. 1 October. https://www.who.int/news-room/feature-stories/detail/a-virus-that-respects-no-borders-protecting-refugees-and-migrants-during-covid-19

WHO (2021). Disability and health. https://www.who.int/en/news-room/fact-sheets/detail/disability-and-health

Worldometer (2021). Coronavirus cases. https://www.worldometers.info/coronavirus/
Yakushko, O. (2009). Xenophobia: Understanding the roots and consequences of negative attitudes toward immigrants. *The Counseling Psychologist, 37*(1), 36–66. https://doi.org/10.1177/0011000008316034
Yuval-Davis, N. (1997). Women, citizenship and difference. *Feminist Review, 57*, 4–27.
Zine, J. (2004). Creating a critical faith-centered space for antiracist feminism: Reflections of a Muslim scholar-activist. *Journal of Feminist Studies in Religion, 20*(2), 167–187. https://doi.org/10.2979/FSR.2004.20.2.167
Zong, J., & Batalova, J. (2017). Syrian refugees in the United States. Migration Policy Institute, 12 January. https://www.migrationpolicy.org/article/syrian-refugees-united-states

Index

abandonment 4, 9, 14, 26, 73
ableism *see also* ableist; xenophobic ableism 2, 51–6, 78, 109
ableist 19–20, 24, 38, 49, 57–8, 87, 110–1, 114
abuse *see also* human rights 4, 16, 21, 39
accepted *see also* gratitude narrative 28, 47, 51, 65, 93, 95
accessibility *see also* mobility; wheelchair use 58–60, 62, 65, 75, 77–85
  adaptive equipment 29, 73, 77, 85, 92–3, 109
  assistive technology 77, 92, 109
  barriers to, 2, 4, 7, 16–22, 28, 35, 38, 44–6, 55–8, 73, 76, 81, 88, 97, 104–14
  challenges 3, 34, 79
  inaccessible 7, 44, 92
accountability 61, 109
action 31, 76, 98, 108–11
actively listening 103–11
Adichie, Chimamanda Ngozi 21–3, 113–5
advocacy 10, 19, 23, 33, 41–2, 44, 47, 53, 89, 93, 95–102, 105, 108–11, 117
Amnesty International Canada 16, 41
amputation 47, 117
anti-colonial *see* colonialism

appropriation 21, 59, 76, 85, 87–9, 94, 104, 110, 115
Arab 1, 3,12, 51, 52, 86, 106
assimilation 1, 4, 49, 68–9, 74–5, 90, 113
asylum 3, 8–10, 23–4, 28, 36, 42, 59, 64–5, 73, 75, 85, 89, 95, 108
  applications 65, 73, 79, 85
  documented 11, 69, 71, 76
  eligibility 78–9
  seekers 23–4, 42
August Reid Institute 52
authentic narratives 42, 63–4, 69

Barbaric Cultural Practices hotline 29
biomedical 18, 38, 41, 44, 47, 54
Blended Visa Office-Referred (BVOR) 8, 13–4
borders 3, 15, 16, 21, 40, 42, 46–8
British Columbia 25

camps *see also* shelters 64, 80
capacity 13, 40, 49, 63, 90
careers *see also* employment; jobs 7, 8, 11, 76–7, 94
caregiver 2, 11, 84, 87
Center for Migration Studies 27
challenges *see* accessibility; children; economic; healthcare
charitable organizations 2, 7, 102

children *see also* education
  challenges 6–9, 78, 81, 87–8, 90–6
  childbirth 59, 97
  childcare 77–78
  paediatrics 2, 61, 86, 116
citizenship 13, 19, 37, 40, 47–49, 55, 114
climate 26, 31, 66, 74, 87
colonialism 1, 5, 18–9, 22–4, 31, 38–9, 43–5, 49–50, 54, 69–70, 91, 111–3
communication 9, 21, 34–5, 38, 77, 82–4, 88–9, 94, 116
  English and American Sign Language (ASL) 89
complex narratives 6
conflict *see also* war 1, 3–4, 9, 12, 15, 31, 39–46, 59–62, 68, 81, 95, 103, 115–6
COVID-19 15–7, 31, 34, 80–1, 88
criminals 24, 35
cultural relevance 1–2, 5, 21, 33, 38, 48–51, 61, 66, 69, 72–3, 88, 95, 106, 113–4

Damascus 7, 33
danger 16, 22, 99, 113
death 4, 15, 17–8, 61, 62
debility 44–7
dehumanizing *see also* 'otherness' 40, 64
diagnoses *see also* misdiagnosis
  acute conditions 29, 59–61, 85
  attention deficit hyperactivity disorder (ADHD) 99–101
  autism spectrum disorder 19
  cerebral palsy 2, 19
  developmental delays 8
  chronic health condition 9
  cognitive 39, 49
  global developmental delay (GDD) 100
  hearing difficulties 83, 89
dignity 28, 58, 67, 91, 100
Director-General WHO 16
disability rights 19, 31, 40–4, 47–8, 54, 85
discrimination *see also* Komagata Maru 4, 28, 32, 47, 51, 52, 54–6, 85, 87–8, 109
disease 16, 47, 59–60, 105, 110
diversity 27, 29, 39, 50, 53, 109
dominant narrative 1, 3, 5, 14, 22–4, 29, 31, 35, 50–1, 61–3, 69, 90, 108, 111–6

economic
  challenges 63, 75–6
  compensation 76
  expenses 13, 76–8, 90
  extreme poverty 5, 62, 65, 105
  financial difficulties 65, 75
  funding 14–5, 78–9, 85–6, 93, 100
  funds 13–5, 78, 85, 97–8
  hardship 1, 4, 16, 63, 115
education *see also* Kumon; Ontario; virtual learning 1, 7–12, 17–9, 25, 28, 65, 69, 76, 82, 85, 89, 92–5, 110
Egypt 8–12, 36, 65
emergency 4, 40, 58–9, 106–7
employment *see also* unemployment; wages 7–11, 28, 48, 52, 65, 75–82, 102, 115

English and American Sign Language (ASL) 89
Environics Institute 52
environment 3, 8, 16, 23, 38, 45, 68, 72–3, 81, 86, 90, 109–11
equality 5, 39, 41
Equity, Diversity, and Inclusion (EDI) 109
ethnicity 15, 25, 27, 48, 51, 115
exclusion 7, 18–20, 24, 32, 39, 43, 47–8, 51, 54–6, 72, 83, 87, 92–4

faith 1, 12, 15, 27, 43, 52, 62, 88, 90–5, 107, 114
family-centred 2, 69, 98, 104–5
federal *see also* Interim Federal Health Program (IFHP) 20, 26, 29, 110
forced displacement 12, 46, 64
forced marriage 8–10
'foreigner' 25, 32, 91
frameworks 18, 24, 32, 37, 42, 110–1
freedom 32, 43, 91
future 6, 8, 9, 60–2, 94, 103, 114–5

Gaza 41, 45, 115–6
gender *see also* women 5, 25, 37, 48, 51, 53–5, 65
genetics 48, 58–60
genocide 45, 116
geopolitical 31, 38
Global North 18–24, 31, 37–45, 49, 50–2, 61, 86, 104, 108–10, 113–6
Global South 22–5, 31, 42–5, 50–1, 104

government 3–4, 12, 13–15, 17, 20, 27–9, 34–5, 42, 70, 77–80, 85, 89, 109
Government-Assisted Refugee (GAR) 13
gratitude narrative *see also* 'welcome' 113

healthcare *see also* biomedical; chronic health condition; Interim Federal Health Program (IFHP); medical; mental health; occupational therapy; World Health Organization (WHO)
  challenges 11, 97–100, 109
  clinics 17–8, 29, 32, 59–60, 63, 68–71, 85, 87, 96–9, 102–7, 111, 116
  culturally responsive care 110
  dental care 86
  doctors 2, 59–61, 70, 85, 89, 91, 97–9, 101, 103–107
  health assessment 110
  hospitals 68–69, 96, 111, 116
  pregnancy 58, 106
  prescriptions 29, 86
  psychiatric hospitals 69
  systems 86, 88
  vaccinations 80
hero narrative 113
hijab *see also* jilbab 2, 23, 32, 87–8, 106–7
history 22, 25, 35, 38, 41, 61, 69, 100–1, 106, 110–1, 116
holistic 33, 102, 110
host country 19, 54, 59, 65–6
housing *see also* shelters 13, 22, 58, 65, 72, 79, 105, 110

human rights *see also* Ontario 4, 16, 31, 37, 39–47, 52, 54, 85–7, 113, 116
humanitarian 4, 10, 12, 15, 19, 24–5, 31, 40, 47, 60

identity 1, 18–9, 39, 46, 51, 57, 62, 103
immigration
   Department of Citizenship and Immigration 19
   Immigration and Refugee Protection Act (IRPA) 25
   Immigration, Refugees and Citizenship Canada (IRCC) 13–14
inclusion 12, 47, 56–7, 83, 85, 92, 94, 109
independence 49, 58, 86, 102
indigenous 29, 31, 41, 45, 55, 69, 91
influence 22–3, 24, 41–2, 53, 114
intergenerational 44, 69, 70, 110
Interim Federal Health Program (IFHP) 29
international law 28, 40
intersectional 32, 39, 51–6, 65, 69, 89, 96, 102, 106–10, 113–4
interviews 11, 18–9, 32, 34, 80, 84, 108
Islamophobia 2, 31, 51–5
isolation 72, 81, 84, 87, 93, 102

jilbab 87, 114
jobs *see also* careers; employment 1, 28, 62–3, 76
Jordan 7, 8, 10–2, 65

justice 4, 39, 42–9, 53–4, 61, 69, 91, 113

Komagata Maru 25
Kumon 98

learning 9, 35, 58–9, 66, 81–4, 88–9, 94–5, 98, 101, 103
Lebanon 9, 10, 12, 60, 65–6
listening *see also* actively listening 5, 33, 97, 103–5, 107
literacy 1, 5, 22, 25, 48, 97
living conditions 16, 50, 85, 91

maimed *see also* amputation; mass disablement 45, 61
malnutrition 4, 116
Mardini sisters 23–4
marginalized 2, 15–7, 21, 26, 30, 43, 80, 108, 115
marriage *see* forced marriage
media 1, 3–5, 13, 17, 22–3, 25–9, 52–3, 63, 66, 116–7
medical *see also* biomedical; healthcare
   history 110
   medication 58–60, 96, 99
   professionals 58, 81, 105
   records 104
mental health 68, 70, 81, 93
methodology 32–4
middle-class 25, 49, 54–5
migration *see also* Center for Migration Studies 1, 10, 21, 27, 37, 42–9, 54, 64–8, 95, 115
military 31, 46, 58, 60, 96, 116
misdiagnoses 104–5

mistreatment 28, 64, 69
mobility 9, 65
Muslim *see also* Islamophobia 1–2, 7, 23–6, 32, 43, 52, 67, 87–90, 106–8

narratives *see* authentic narratives; complex narratives; dominant narrative; gratitude narrative; hero narrative; Mardini sisters
newcomers 28, 51, 75, 109, 117
non-disabled 4, 25, 38, 44, 49–50, 94–5
non-dominant stories 6, 22–3, 69, 117
'normal' 20, 38, 48–9, 106

occupation *see also* careers; employment; jobs 2, 36, 39, 95, 115
occupational therapy 2, 69, 97–8
Ontario 1, 18, 23, 33, 54, 59, 69, 93–4
  Ford, Doug 17, 93
  Public Health Ontario 18
  Human Rights Commission 54
  Ministry of Education 94
oppression 2, 39, 43, 47, 52–6, 69, 72, 90, 103, 109–13
'otherness' 37, 74, 91, 114

pandemic 15–17, 31, 80–4
parents *see also* children 1, 19, 58, 77, 82, 84, 87–8, 90–2, 97, 104
participation 2, 5, 43, 47–9, 77, 93

persecution 3, 5, 20–1, 27, 43, 65
police 32, 35–6, 43, 50, 53
policies 5, 15–16, 19, 21–30, 38–9, 42–3, 48, 52, 55, 77, 87, 108–11, 114
policymakers 32, 111, 114
populations 17, 26, 32, 38, 41, 45, 69–70, 80, 99, 108, 117
post-9/11 27, 43
poverty 1, 5, 10, 48, 62, 65–6, 96, 105, 110
power 14, 21–29, 31, 33–5, 39, 41–2, 50, 54, 91, 105–7, 111, 113–4
Prime Minister Justin Trudeau 3, 27–8
private sponsorship 8, 9, 12–5, 22, 108
privilege *see also* supremacist 28, 31–5, 43, 55, 96
protection 16, 20, 24–5, 27–8, 40, 43, 58, 71, 116–7
protocols 16, 32, 61, 80, 88
psychological 44, 62–3, 72, 96, 99, 110, 115
public spaces 4, 17, 43, 52, 91
public transport 74–5

Quebec 31–2, 43
Quran 90, 95

racialized 2, 17, 22–7, 31, 36, 43–5, 51, 55, 88, 110
racism *see also* discrimination; supremacists 2–3, 25, 30–1, 51, 54–5, 87, 111, 114
reflections 34, 63, 69, 113, 115, 117

refugee *see also* Syria
  Convention 1951 28
  crisis 3, 11–2, 24–5, 113
  status 9
rehabilitation 73, 86, 111
religion *see also* faith 17, 27, 43
resettlement 4, 10, 12, 13–4, 24–6, 66, 73, 88, 90, 95
resilience 1, 96, 117
resources 3, 13–5, 26, 29, 50, 56, 65, 73, 79, 81–8, 90–1, 94, 98, 100, 109–10
respite 77, 82, 85
rights *see* disability rights; human rights; United Nation (UN)

safeguarding 9, 11, 17, 27, 40, 62, 68, 73, 81, 90, 103, 109–11, 115
Said, Edward 50
sanctions 31, 46, 58, 60, 96, 115
schools *see also* education 1, 17, 19, 31, 43, 52, 66, 69–70, 77, 93, 116
security 1, 27, 36, 41, 43, 52, 62, 65, 110, 115
sensory 39, 70, 94
service providers 2, 32, 70, 105, 110
settlement 11, 26, 70–3, 76, 79, 92, 103, 109
'settler-colonial' 19, 22, 43, 69–70, 91, 111, 113
shelters *see also* temporary shelter 17, 29, 91–2
slavery 45, 69
SMILE Canada 2, 71, 79, 87, 95
social
  activists 18
  conditions 5, 39, 75
  determinants 4, 38, 69, 102, 110, 113
  justice 4, 39, 113
  media 3, 22, 26, 116–7
  Model of Refugeehood
  services 1–2, 17, 19, 85, 102
  welfare 29, 48
socializing 9, 58
socioeconomic 17, 31, 48
sociopolitical 1, 31, 39
sponsorship *see also* private sponsorship 7, 8, 9, 12–5, 22, 75, 108
sponsorship agreement holders (SAH) 12
stigma 58, 88
stories *see also* narratives
  'single story' 22–3, 31
  storytelling 5, 21, 32–4, 113, 117
supremacists 35, 52
Syria 6–12, 15–6, 23, 26, 33, 40, 46, 58–66, 70–7, 81, 87–9, 99, 103–4, 113
  Operation Syrian Refugees 12
  Syrian refugee crisis 3, 11–2, 24–5, 113
systemic *see also* debility
  barriers 4, 18, 38–9, 56, 106–7
  change 28, 114

teachers *see also* education; schools 32, 58, 79, 82–4, 88–9, 92–4, 103
temporary shelter 29, 91–2
theoretical 20, 37, 44, 57, 114–5
threats 27, 42, 51, 65, 80
Toronto 3, 27, 29, 85

torture 4, 16, 116
transnational intersectionality 54–5
trauma 4, 21, 44, 46, 62–3, 68–72, 81, 96, 103, 105, 110–6
Trump, Donald 3, 25–6, 51,
'truths' 1, 5, 21–2, 115
Türkiye 12, 65

UN Secretary-General 15
'undeserving' 2, 37, 39, 58, 108
unemployment 48, 62
United Nation (UN)
    Convention on the Rights of Persons with Disabilities (CRPD) 39–41
    Department of Economic and Social Affairs (UNDESA) 21
    Leaders' Summit on Refugees 28
    UNHCR 12–7, 28
United States *see also* Trump, Donald 3, 25–6, 29, 35, 41, 45, 52–3, 71
'unsanitary' 7, 16, 80, 117
Vancouver 25

violations 16, 39, 43, 47
violence *see also* weapons 1, 5, 12, 27, 44–7, 51–3, 57, 71, 96, 103–5, 113–5
virtual learning 34, 81–4, 88
volunteers 13–4, 75, 92
vulnerable 12, 15, 21, 22, 24, 50, 65, 80, 85, 108, 117

wages 76–7
war 7–12, 23–7, 43–6, 49, 57–64, 66, 69, 100–3, 115
'war on terror' *see also* post-9/11 26, 43
weapons 44, 61, 99, 116–7
weather *see* climate
'welcome' 25–9
well-being 2, 8, 30, 56, 59–60, 68, 78, 83–6, 99, 106, 111, 115–7
wheelchair use 7, 57
women 15, 26, 41–3, 53, 61, 71, 95
Women's Refugee Committee 4
World Health Organization (WHO) 15–6

xenophobic ableism 2, 51–6

www.ingramcontent.com/pod-product-compliance
Lightning Source LLC
Chambersburg PA
CBHW071714020426
42333CB00017B/2259